I0500515

Help Your Chronic Condition Nightmare

Barry A. Coniglio Jr. D.C., D.A.B.C.O., F.A.C.O., C.C.S.P.

ISBN: 1463740506

ISBN 13: 978-1463740504

DEDICATION

To my family, for giving me life and for showing me how to live it in balance. I am truly grateful for your gifts of love, humility and compassion.

Thank you for fueling my soul and giving me the validation I need to continue moving forward. You have taught me life lessons that will always be treasured.

CONTENTS

ACKNOWLEDGMENTS

As with any major project, it takes a great team to make all of the elements come together. I want to extend my sincere thanks to:

My Immediate Family --- They are the best! They know me the best. Thanks for your love and support.

My Office Staff --- It feels good to be involved with a good team. We all have the same goal in mind. That is to help. They amaze me with their dedication to help our patients, community and one another.

Shirley Myers --- My sixth grade English teacher. She taught with excellence. Her lessons sunk in, even though she didn't think so at the time.

Bob Nark --- My high school chemistry teacher who guided and nudged me even when I was an undergraduate college student.

Dr. Dennis Skogsbergh --- The best chiropractic orthopedic professor I have come across. He taught with such confidence, which stays with me today.

Dr. Mike Johnson --- My teacher of brain based therapy. His program of instruction helped integrate the neurological based treatment with my chiropractic, orthopedic and physical techniques.

W. A. Boyer --- I am grateful to my editor, W. A. Boyer, for his hard work and careful attention with this piece.

FOREWORD

It is a great honor to introduce the author of this book to you. I have been a friend and colleague of Dr. Barry Coniglio for nearly twenty years and have developed a tremendous respect for his dedication to his patients, his community, as well as to his profession. It is no surprise that he has chosen to author this compilation on chronic conditions because he has spent his career dedicated to expertly treating those suffering with both acute and chronic issues.

Today we are inundated with information, some beneficial and some detrimental, regarding a multitude of health issues. All one has to do is watch late night television infomercials, read some advertising, or simply open the "junk" mail. How is one to know what information we can trust? The only way to truly know is to trust the source. The book you are about to read will inform those of you suffering with a variety of chronic conditions that there are options available to you that can safely and effectively help improve your life and restore your health.

Dr. Coniglio has spent many years studying natural methods to assist the body in restoration of health.   He has earned his Doctor of Chiropractic degree from the Los Angeles College of Chiropractic. He then has continued his educational pursuits by becoming a Board Certified Chiropractic Sports Physician as well as becoming a Board Certified Chiropractic Orthopedist. Additionally he has extensive education in nutrition, rehabilitation, and neurologic disorders.

It is this degree of educational commitment that qualifies him to author this text regarding chronic conditions.

Dr. Stanley Piltin D.C., F.A.C.O..

Dr. Coniglio has been a friend and colleague for over ten years. The first thing that comes to mind is his positive energy.

He has built a very successful chiropractic wellness practice in Southern New Jersey. Dr. Coniglio combines both the clinical expertise with excellent personal communication skills. He is constantly researching new ways to help and convey the chiropractic health message to the public, both internally in his office and externally in the community. He is always evolving both professionally and personally.

The best compliment I can give my friend, Barry, is that I wouldn't have achieved the success I enjoy without his leadership, encouragement and support.

Gerald J Agasar DC
Partner in The Wellness Solution Centers
121 Friends lane Suite 100
Newtown, Pa. 18940

Help Your Chronic Condition Nightmare

INTRODUCTION

Ask yourself the following questions:

How has your chronic condition affected your relationships, finances, family, or other activities? What has it cost you in time, money, happiness, sleep? Where do you picture yourself in the next one to three years if your condition is not taken care of soon? What is it worth to you if we could improve your condition?

Good health means to experience the peace of mind, meaning and value in life which allow us to cope with the challenges we face. It turns out that people who experience a high quality of life have a stronger immune system, are sick less and have shorter illness by disease than people who do not experience life as good and meaningful.

My mission as a physician is to help you achieve peace of mind and assist you in finding value in life through treating your illness and lessening your pain. We all face challenges as our lives evolve, and my mission is to help you achieve self-actualization and be as happy and healthy as possible.

This book was written for you. If you are suffering, in pain or ill, it is my hope this book will be a vehicle leading to the knowledge and understanding that you can change things. Here, I strive to present that knowledge to you.

Help Your Chronic Condition Nightmare

Legal Disclaimer

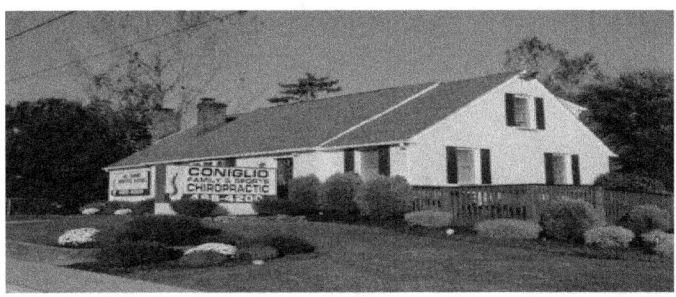

The medical treatments and therapies described in this book are not intended to replace the services of a trained health professional. Your personal physical condition and diagnosis may require specific individualized modifications or precautions. Before undertaking any form of treatment, therapy or starting exercise, you should consult your physician or licensed health care provider. Any repercussions from the application of ideas, suggestions or procedures set forth in this book are the reader's sole responsibility.

The trademarks, service marks, logos and devices displayed are the exclusive property of Dr. Barry A. Coniglio Jr. and are protected under U.S. and various international jurisdictional trademark and copyright laws. Use of any of these instruments without prior express written consent from the author is strictly prohibited.

The design, images, text and overall layout are protected under U.S. and international law as copyrighted materials. Anyone who claims, displays, reproduces copies or creates derivative works for commercial or non-commercial purposes without the prior written consent from the author is in violation of copyright laws and will be held liable for copyright infringement under the relevant jurisdictions.

Help Your Chronic Condition Nightmare

Chapter One

The Awakening

There are a couple of incidents in my life that crafted desires and provided meaningful insight which lead me to the career path I now excel in. It's much more than a vocation because I am humbled to be able to use the unique birthright gifts passed on to me. For me, this meant finding the common thread in the things I knew I was good at and really wanted to do that made a positive difference in the lives of others, it meant incorporating the things that I was honestly passionate about and felt uniquely suited for into my life. This allows me to help others and make the world itself a better place in which to be. It is these events which fueled my true passion and helped seat my calling.

In my high school days, my beloved grandfather had lung cancer. I've always been very close with my family and I experienced firsthand the different types of suffering my grandfather went through before he finally passed away at the age of sixty-five. The medical community does its best in the treatment of cancer. Overall, the medical community has made outstanding leaps in research and is many times successful at prolonging peoples' lives who are victims of this horrible, life threatening and devastating illness. My grandfather, like many other people who have this horrible disease, did suffer at times through the chemotherapy designed to help make him better. It was devastating to watch and stand by while this once strong man got eaten away by

1

the cells of his own body – and then the cure, which became a curse, made him sicker.

That is when I really became interested in the health field. I truly wanted to help people on a personal level. Sometimes it seems physicians can become numb to their patient's problems and sufferings: I watched it happen. It was then I knew I wanted to approach some level of health care as a vocation, but in a different manner and with a more humanistic approach to my bedside manner and treatment. I knew it would take years of hard work and study, but it was then I knew I wanted to become a physician.

What sparked my interest in chiropractic health was when I played baseball for Gloucester Catholic High School in New Jersey. I was athletic back in high school, but not one of the more standout baseball players on the team. I was surrounded by outstanding talent, but I did manage to hold my own.

During one game, right in the middle of the season, I remember the pitcher pitched a pitch right down the middle of the plate! Absolutely perfect - no movement on it… a perfect homerun ball; or so I thought. It actually was a strikeout ball. I swung the bat as hard as I could and completely missed the ball. I also wrenched my lower back. I had to do something for the pain so I went to the family medical doctor whose treatment of choice back then was to give me anti-inflammatory medication in combination with muscle relaxers.

The muscle relaxers made me so tired that I ended up missing one entire week of school lying flat on my back because of the effects of the muscle relaxer combined with a newly found bad back. The muscle relaxer made me so drowsy that I could hardly walk, much less function as a student. Even now I can't see how patients in chronic pain function when enduring the sometimes bad side effects of a muscle relaxer. Why live life like a zombie? Unfortunately, a lot of people are on these meds and they tend to stay on them for a long time believing it's their only choice of real relief.

After a week of this, I called a local chiropractor by the name of Dr. James Tighe, and went to see him. He still is very personable and down-to-earth - the kind of fellow you automatically can't help but like when you first meet him. He performed an initial examination and an x-ray. He took time with me, found the exact cause of my pain, and explained to me in words I understood about his treatment approach. It only took a few short visits to his office with chiropractic and physiotherapy treatment, and I was back on the baseball field. We did win the South Jersey Championship by the way, but we lost in the state finals. Honestly, I was just happy to be able to get back on the field as soon as possible thanks to Dr. Tighe's care and treatment.

The third event which literally helped me decide to explore the profession of chiropractic was that I also played football. I remember vividly that in between my junior and senior season, I was exercising, working out lifting weights with a good friend of mine, Steven McDermott. We fed off of each other's motivation and goals, so we worked out three times a week. Steven was not able to play football in his sophomore year due to an injury to his knee, and then knee surgery to repair the injury.

After his sophomore year and his knee surgery, Steve played sparingly as a junior due to his nagging, still constantly bothersome knee injury. It was the summer in between our junior and senior playing seasons that someone

3

recommended that he go and see a chiropractor. I drove at the time and he did not, so he asked me to drive him to his appointment, which I gladly did and I observed the treatment from this particular chiropractor.

Now, this chiropractor treated my friend a little bit differently than my chiropractor treated me. Tests showed empirically that the primary reason Steve's knee was not able to be balanced, stabilized, and grow strong again was because of an adrenal gland insufficiency and the stress related to that specific gland. Steve's treatment was dietary in nature. This particular chiropractor recommended that Steven drink no caffeine and not eat any foods that had sugar in it whatsoever. This treatment lasted for three months – and it worked. As a result, Steven was able to play football his senior year with minimal knee pain and had a very successful football season. This was an epiphany moment and I knew right then and there what I wanted to do in my life.

Preparation

In my senior year of high school, I realized due to my personal experiences combined with my friends personal successful chiropractic treatments that I wanted to become a chiropractor. I attended Glassboro State College in New Jersey and took the necessary science courses with a grade point average of a 3.8 and matriculated to Los Angles College of Chiropractic. Los Angles College of Chiropractic was a very difficult school, but it prepared me for my dream of becoming a chiropractor. I started Chiropractic College in January 1986 and completed in April 1989. This course work was year round without summers off. That is equivalent to a five year program but I decided to complete the course work without taking summer breaks.

After graduating with a chiropractic degree in 1989, I matriculated to New York Chiropractic College and became a board certified chiropractic sports physician. That was completed in 1990. In 1992, I matriculated to National College of Chiropractic in Lombard, Illinois for a four year program in chiropractic orthopedics. In 1998, I completed all of the prescribed orthopedic examinations which were oral and written and became a board certified chiropractic orthopedist.

I was fortunate to pass my boards on the first try and then my life got a bit easier. Not missing those three to four hours of constant studying each night for one straight year, I was able to relax a little bit and really concentrate on helping the patient's in my office. Our office became very, very busy from that point on and we started to get completely booked with appointments. That made me feel really good because I knew we were helping a lot of people. My chiropractic team has been very dedicated. They put our patient's lives and care first. Our office staff is exceptional and dedicated. We have stuck together for a long period of time and our motto is "service to the patient first".

Coniglio Chiropractic Wellness Center is a modern facility known for its vast range of chiropractic techniques, care and other services. Here, we treat the whole person, not just a symptom. We offer:

✓ Chiropractic Family Care

✓ Acupuncture

✓ Sports Chiropractic

✓ Massage Therapy

- ✓ Low-Level Laser Treatment

- ✓ Computerized Nerve Scan Technology

- ✓ Wellness Workshops

- ✓ Physiotherapy

- ✓ Therapeutic Exercise Rehab

- ✓ Computerized Foot/Arch Scanning and Orthotics

- ✓ Whole-food Nutritional Supplementation

- ✓ Meditation Instruction

We believe in the power of natural healing, so much so that we have devoted our lives to building and promoting it. You could say we're now experts at it. We specialize in chiropractic care for the whole family, acupuncture, and sports related chiropractic medicine; massage therapy along with low-level laser treatments. We offer computerized nerve scan technology, optimal wellness seminars to the public, physiotherapy, therapeutic exercise rehabilitation; computerized foot and arch orthotics, nutritional supplement recommendations, training and guidance, meditation instruction, metabolic and neurological testing and treatment – and more!

Our office has never been a cookie-cutter operation, it's very unique. We are very specific and tend to the needs of every patient. Because life evolves and needs change, we have the ability to change treatment plans from visit to visit until we find what works for the patient, especially with our most difficult, chronic, and severe patients. Many facilities I know setup a treatment and plan and treat three times a week for a four week period of time and regardless of how well that patient progresses, or does not progress they stick to that treatment plan. Not us, if we find something that benefits the patient more, we change gears if we need to. Actually, our office changes gears all the time, and it's because we take time to listen to the patient and then act on what we hear.

Testimonial

Patient: Susan L. Fean

Chief Complaint Treated: Post-Surgical Spinal Stenosis, 2 Herniated Discs

After suffering from severe back pain for years, my primary doctor recommended an MRI. The results showed 2 herniated discs. He suggested I see my neurologist at a renowned hospital in Philadelphia. The (recommended) course of treatment was to have back surgery.

This relieved the pain for about 2 months, then scar tissue developed and the pain was back. I was sent for steroid injections (3 sessions!) – The pain was still there. I then went to Pain Management and was given medication and since I am allergic to morphine, I had an allergic reaction to the medication; so the medication I could take was not strong enough.

I couldn't get out of bed in the morning without pain; I had to walk along the wall and hang on to the furniture until I could straighten out or walk without discomfort. Lying in bed and trying to turn over was difficult – I had to grab on to the headboard and turn my body: This after having surgery and injections. The bottom line was I was no better off than before I had the surgery.

My primary doctor told me I (had) two options left and that was chiropractic treatment or to have an implant for pain. I decided to try chiropractic treatments. I was the biggest skeptic going into this. I really did not think it would work.

I started my treatment in 2003. My treatments began with daily sessions, then (went down to) 3 times a week, then twice a week; then weekly; monthly and now I'm down to every 6 weeks. I really did not think it would help! I'm at the point (now) where I can get out of bed without pain and am able to do things I couldn't do like vacuuming, yard work and walking. It's been a long haul but I've literally gotten my life back to where it should be. I still have flair ups, but with treatment it doesn't last long.

Chapter Two

Chronic Conditions

As licensed health care professionals concerned with the analysis, management and prevention of chronic disorders - and the havoc these disorders cause on the general health and in the lives of our patients, we test and treat our patients metabolically, neurologically and physically. We use every diagnostic tool at our disposal: biochemistry, microbiology, pathology, anatomy, physiology, diagnostic sciences and more. We analyze the unique role played by the proper functioning of these vast systems verses what you as an individual now experience, and we bring the body as a whole back into homeostasis. Homeostasis is when the body functions as it should with each body system working in unison and complementing each other. We leave no stone unturned in determining the absolute cause of your condition – and if we can, we fix it – period.

While all conditions and ailments directly affect your life, some wreak more havoc than others. People tend to suffer from many of the same health problems in general simply because the human body tends to react the same way for many people, but because you are unique – you as a person require individualized treatment. Let's take a look at some of the more common ailments we see and have experience in successfully treating.

Fibromyalgia: More than 12 million people in this country suffer from fibromyalgia and most are women in the age group between 25 and 60 years old. Women are eight to ten times

9

more likely to suffer from this sometimes crippling disease than are men. Fibromyalgia is a condition which causes your whole body to ache and sometimes, throb.

Some people suffer crippling fatigue -- even upon arising fresh from a long nights sleep. Sometimes, it feels like the condition will never go away. Many times, muscles twitch, burn, or have a very deep stabbing pain sensation. Specific tender points on the body may be literally painful to touch, so people with this condition tend to avoid situations which solicit tactile stimulation. In addition there may be swelling, disturbances in deep-level or restful sleep, and mood disturbances or depression accordingly. Fibromyalgia can cause feelings similar to osteoarthritis, bursitis, and tendinitis in that deep aches or soreness you can't get rid of is present. Fibromyalgia problems can include bad headaches, irritable-bowel syndrome, irritable bladder, cognitive Fibro-fog and memory problems from inescapable pain along with restless leg syndrome, an acute sensitivity to noise and temperature and more.

When your life gets turned upside down, it can have a negative impact on others lives as well. Fibromyalgia victims sometimes find it difficult to maintain existing friendships, relationships or even meet new people. Due to a lack of complete medical understanding about the condition as a whole, your loved ones may find themselves becoming frustrated with people experiencing fibromyalgia. The emotional turmoil and physical pain associated with this condition --as well as some of the medications used to treat it--also can lower an individual's sex drive, desire or motivation, straining intimate relationships sometimes to the breaking point.

Through training, experience and compassion, I have learned I can help people with fibromyalgia lead normal and productive lives.

Peripheral Neuropathy (PN): Peripheral neuropathy is a medical term describing the damage to the peripheral nervous system - the nerves that run to the arms and legs.

Over one hundred types of peripheral neuropathy have been identified so far, each type with its own unique characteristic set of signs and symptoms, patterns of development, and unique prognosis. Specific function and symptoms are dependent on the type of nerves involved – motor nerves, sensory nerves, or autonomic nerves. Some folks may experience provisional numbness, minor or major tingling sensations, a "pricking" sensation; sensitivity to touch is common as is muscle weakness. Other people may suffer more intense symptoms; those include a burning pain particularly at night while laying down, acute muscle wasting, partial paralysis, or systemic organ or gland dysfunction. Peripheral neuropathy is either inherited or acquired.

The causes of acquired peripheral neuropathy incorporate physical injury, trauma to a nerve or branch, some tumors, many toxins, human autoimmune responses, nutritional deficiencies have been linked as has alcoholism, and many identified vascular and metabolic disorders. Acquired peripheral neuropathies can be caused by systemic disease process, some form of trauma from external or outside agents and infections or autoimmune disorders which affect nerve tissue. Inherited forms of peripheral neuropathy are caused by inborn anomalies in the genetic coding during fetal development or by genetic mutations.

While no cure exists for inherited peripheral neuropathy, there are therapies which we provide that can help you live as normal life as possible. We can help you adopt healthy habits -- like maintaining optimal weight, avoid exposure to toxins, and following a physician-supervised program of exercise. Because we emphasize a holistic approach, things like eating a specific diet, identifying vitamin deficiencies, and limiting or completely avoiding alcohol can reduce the physical and emotional effects.

Diabetic Peripheral Neuropathy: Diabetic peripheral neuropathy is a nerve disorder caused by diabetes or which is related to poor blood sugar control. The most common types of diabetic peripheral neuropathy can result in problems with sensation of the feet. It generally develops slowly after several years of living with diabetes but may occur early in the disease in some cases. The symptoms are a feeling of general numbness, pain or tingling in the feet or lower legs. The pain can be quite intense and require treatment to relieve the discomfort. The loss of sensation in the feet may also increase the possibility that foot injuries will go unnoticed and develop into ulcers or lesions that become infected. In some cases, diabetic peripheral neuropathy can be associated with difficulty walking and weakness in the muscles of the feet.

There are other types of diabetic-related neuropathies that affect specific parts of the body. For example, diabetic amyotrophy; a degeneration of the muscles caused by nerve disease that causes pain, weakness and the literal wasting of certain muscles, or cranial nerve blockages that can result in double vision eyesight, a drooping eyelid, or dizziness. Diabetes can also affect the autonomic nerves that control blood pressure, the digestive tract, bladder function, and sexual organs. Problems with the autonomic nerves may cause lightheadedness, indigestion, diarrhea or constipation, difficulty with bladder control, and impotence.

The goal of treating diabetic peripheral neuropathy is to prevent further tissue damage and relieve discomfort. The first step is to bring blood sugar levels under control. Another important part of treatment involves taking special care of the feet by wearing proper fitting shoes and routinely checking the feet for cuts and infections. Some individuals find that walking regularly, taking warm baths, or using elastic stockings may help relieve leg pain.

The prognosis for diabetic peripheral neuropathy depends largely on how well the underlying condition of diabetes is handled. That's why you need someone with experience in treating this disorder. Treating the diabetes may halt progression and improve symptoms of peripheral neuropathy.

Thyroid Dysfunction: The thyroid gland is a small gland located in the front of the neck. It is made up of two halves; each half called a lobe and connected by a narrow band of tissue. The function of the thyroid gland is to take iodine and convert it into thyroid hormones: thyroxine or T4 and triiodothyronine or T3.

The thyroid is unique because thyroid cells are the only cells in the body which can absorb iodine taken in by the food we eat. These cells combine iodine and the amino acid tyrosine to make T3 and T4. T3 and T4 are then released into the blood stream and are transported throughout the body where they control metabolism – the conversion of oxygen and calories to energy. Every cell in the body depends on thyroid hormones for regulation of their metabolism.

The thyroid gland is under the control of the pituitary gland, a small gland the size of a peanut at the base of the brain. When the level of thyroid hormones drops too low, the pituitary gland produces something called Thyroid Stimulating Hormone or TSH, that kick-starts the thyroid gland to produce more hormones. It's easier to imagine the thyroid gland as a furnace and the pituitary gland as the thermostat of the body working in conjunction with one another.

When thyroid dysfunction occurs, it can wreak chaos inside the body. Because the function of the thyroid gland is to regulate the speed of the body's metabolism and convert the food we eat into energy, when this gland is not operating properly it causes all kinds of problems in the body. The effects of those problems are immediate and sometimes acute, because the chemical balance of the body is thrown off. That chemical imbalance; also known as a hormone imbalance, affects other body organs and thus body systems.

Thyroid hormones control metabolism and organ function and directly affect weight loss or gain, energy levels, skin condition, heart rate, cholesterol levels, menstrual regularity and memory along with other body functions. When not enough thyroid hormone is produced, a condition called hypothyroidism will result, often referred to as an underactive thyroid.

Because there are so many different health problems associated with either an underactive or overactive thyroid gland, it is essential that basic thyroid function be tested regularly and if needed, definitive action taken to correct the problems accordingly. Common symptoms of thyroid dysfunction are directly related to hormone imbalance. They can include:

- The feeling of cold hands and feet
- Forgetfulness, dementia
- Constipation
- Weight gain
- Depression
- High cholesterol
- Dry or coarse skin
- Fatigue and weakness
- Hair loss
- Sleep difficulties
- Heavy menstrual periods
- Immune system problems
- Nervousness, tremors

Follow the guidance of a qualified natural practitioner for the natural treatment of thyroid dysfunction and in most cases they can help you lead a normal, happy life with minimal stress or effort on your part.

Insomnia and Lack of Sleep: Insomnia, also known as sleep deprivation, is a common condition in which you have trouble falling or staying asleep leading to lack of sleep over time. This condition can range from mild to severe, depending on how often it occurs and for how long it lingers. Insomnia can cause excessive daytime sleepiness and a lack of energy. It also can make you feel anxious, depressed, or irritable. You may have trouble focusing on tasks, paying attention, learning, and remembering. This can make simple things like driving dangerous. It can cause mistakes at work and many times, job performance suffers.

Sleep deprivation is getting more and more common in our stressed-out society. Nine out of ten people of the working population would sleep longer in the morning if they had the chance, and almost one third of the population suffer from sleep deprivation. About ten percent of the population is constantly getting too little sleep. Half of these cases are due to problems falling asleep and the other half are due to disturbances by, for example, children or noise. Insomnia is more common with women than men.

Insomnia can be chronic or acute. Chronic insomnia is classified as symptoms occurring at least 3 nights a week for more than one month. Acute insomnia lasts for less time. Some people who have insomnia may have trouble falling asleep. Other people may fall asleep easily but wake up too soon. Others may have trouble with both falling asleep and staying asleep. As a result, insomnia may cause you to get too little sleep or have poor-quality sleep. You may not feel refreshed or rested when you wake up. This can adversely affect various parts of your life.

Sleep is divided into five stages and when you pass through all five stages, you start all over at stage one. One such sequence is called a sleep cycle. Here follows a short description of the five stages of sleep:

You get drowsy. Your heart rate slows down, you start to breathe slower and your metabolism slows down. This stage usually lasts five to twenty minutes.

You enter light sleep: This type of sleep constitutes about half of the total sleep time.

You enter the two stages of deep sleep: During these stages the brain activity is at its lowest. The body produces almost no stress hormones but a lot of growth hormones.

Dream sleep, also known as REM sleep: During this stage the eyes are moving rapidly behind the eyelids, hence the name Rapid Eye Movement or REM. During this stage breathing gets faster, the heart beats a little faster and your blood pressure rises. The brain now works in a similar way as when we are awake. You can dream during all stages of sleep, but dreams are most common during this stage.

There are two types of insomnia; primary and secondary.

While primary insomnia is less common, it is not caused by a medical problem, medicines, or other substances and is classified as an entity all its own. A number of life-changes can trigger primary insomnia, including long-lasting stress and emotional upset. The most common type is called secondary insomnia. This type of insomnia is a symptom or side effect of some other preexisting problem. More than 8 out of 10 people suffer from secondary insomnia.

There seems to be a connection between long term sleep problems and cardiovascular diseases and depression. Sleep deprivation caused by insomnia lowers the immune defense and can cause heightened sensitivity to pain, which can worsen the symptoms of pain diseases like fibromyalgia and arthritis. This can also be a factor behind elevated blood pressure. Sleep in itself has a reducing effect on blood pressure and with too little sleep the body's ability to regulate blood pressure is reduced.

I have a high success rate in helping those suffering from lack of sleep. I can literally get you dreaming again!

Restless Leg Syndrome: Restless leg syndrome or RLS for short is a common cause of painful, tired legs. The leg pain of restless leg syndrome typically eases with motion of the legs and becomes more noticeable at rest. Restless leg syndrome also features worsening of symptoms and leg pain during the early evening or later at night. RLS is classified as a movement disorder because individuals are forced to move their legs in order to gain relief from symptoms.

The most distinctive or unusual aspect of the condition is that lying down and trying to relax activates the symptoms and seems to make the symptoms more pronounced. Most people with RLS have difficulty falling asleep and when they fall asleep, staying asleep. If left untreated, the condition causes exhaustion and daytime fatigue. Many people with Restless Leg Syndrome report that their job, personal relations, and activities of daily living are strongly affected as a result of their sleep deprivation. They are often unable to concentrate, have impaired memory, or fail to accomplish daily tasks because they are so tired. It also can make traveling difficult and can cause depression.

RLS occurs in both men and women, although the incidence is about twice as high in the female population. It may begin at any age. Many individuals who are severely affected are middle-aged or older, and the symptoms typically become more frequent and last longer with age.

People with RLS feel uncomfortable sensations in their legs, especially when sitting or lying down, accompanied by an irresistible urge to move the affected limb. These sensations less commonly affect the arms, trunk, or head of the body. Although the sensations can occur on just one side of the body, they most often affect both sides.

Because moving the legs relieves the discomfort, people with Restless Leg Syndrome often keep their legs in motion to minimize or prevent the sensations. They may pace the floor, constantly move their legs while sitting, and toss and turn in bed.

A classic feature of RLS is that the symptoms are worse at night with a distinct symptom-free period in the early morning, allowing for more refreshing sleep at that time. Other triggering situations are periods of inactivity such as long car trips, sitting in a movie theater, long-distance flights, immobilization in a cast, or relaxation exercises. Many individuals also note a worsening of symptoms if their sleep is further reduced by events or activity.

RLS symptoms may vary from day to day and in severity and frequency from person to person. Individuals with mild RLS may have some disruption of sleep onset and minor interference in daytime activities. In moderately severe cases, symptoms occur only once or twice a week but result in significant delay of sleep onset, with some disruption of daytime function. In severe cases of RLS, the symptoms occur more than twice a week and result in burdensome interruption of sleep and impairment of daytime function.

Individuals with RLS can sometimes experience remissions—spontaneous improvement over a period of weeks or months before symptoms reappear—usually during the early stages of the disorder. In general, however, symptoms become more severe over time.

People who have both RLS and an associated medical condition tend to develop more severe symptoms rapidly. In contrast, those who have RLS that is not related to any other condition and experience onset at an early age show a very slow progression of the disorder; many years may pass before symptoms occur regularly.

In most cases, the cause of RLS is unknown. However, it may have a genetic component; RLS is often found in families where the onset of symptoms is before age 40. Specific gene variants have been associated with RLS. Evidence indicates that low levels of iron in the brain also may be responsible for RLS.

RLS also appears to be related to the following factors or conditions, although researchers do not yet know if these factors actually cause RLS:

Chronic diseases such as kidney failure, diabetes, and peripheral neuropathy. Treating the underlying condition often provides relief from RLS symptoms.

Certain medications that may aggravate symptoms. These medications include antinausea drugs, antipsychotic drugs, antidepressants that increase serotonin (a chemical which allows electricity to flow through the body), and some cold and allergy medications that contain sedating antihistamines.

Pregnancy, especially in the last trimester. In most cases, symptoms usually disappear within 4 weeks after delivery.

Alcohol and sleep deprivation also may aggravate or trigger symptoms in some individuals. Because I have successfully treated many individuals who suffer from this horrible condition, I am well aware of what it takes to bring you the relief you so desperately seek.

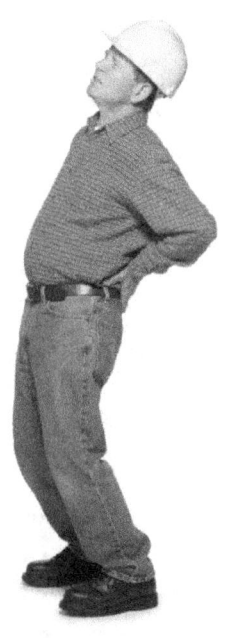

Herniated, Bulging or Degenerative Disc: I'm no stranger to chronic back pain – pain that just never seems to go away. When I played baseball, I learned firsthand about this condition. To herniate means to bulge or stick out. Discs of the spine are really the soft cushions in between the bones of the spine. A herniated disc is a displaced fragment of the center, called the nucleus that is pushed through a tear in the outer layer of the disc.

Often when a disc is herniated, it is in the early stages of degeneration or in a declining phase from its normal healthy state. Herniated discs are common in the lumbar spine, a part of the backbone that is between the bottom of the ribs and hips.

Activity, stress or injury often cause herniated discs. A herniated disc may even be caused by a single excessive strain. The firmness and sharp pain a person feels down the leg because of the slipped disk is called sciatica. People who are 30 to 40 years of age are most commonly affected by herniated discs. Research shows that a predisposition for slipped discs may occur in families, often affecting several family members.

As we age, our spinal discs break down, or degenerate. As the space between the vertebrae gets smaller, there is less padding between them, and the spine becomes less stable. These age-related changes include:

The loss of fluid in your discs. This reduces the ability of the discs to act as shock absorbers and makes them less flexible. Loss of fluid also makes the disc thinner and narrows the distance between the vertebrae.

Tiny tears or cracks in the outer layer of the disc. The jellylike material inside the disc may be forced out through the tears or cracks, which cause the discs to bulge, break open or rupture, or even break into fragments.

This may result in back or neck pain, but this varies from person to person. Many people have no pain, while others with the same amount of disc damage have severe pain that limits their activities. Where the pain occurs depends on the location of the affected disc. An affected disc in the neck area may result in neck or arm pain, while an affected disc in the lower back may result in pain in the back, buttocks, or leg. The pain often gets worse with movements such as bending over, reaching up, or twisting.

The pain may start after a major injury such as from a car accident, a minor injury such as a fall from a low height or an old football injury, or something as simple as a normal motion such as bending over to pick something up. It may also start gradually for no known reason and get worse over time.

Diagnosing this condition starts with asking about your symptoms, past injuries or illnesses, any previous treatment you may have had, and your habits and activities that may be causing pain in the neck, arms, back, buttocks, or legs. During the physical examination, some of the things that must be evaluated are:

* the affected area's range of motion and for pain caused by movement;

* areas of tenderness and any nerve-related changes, such as numbness, tingling, or weakness in the affected area, or changes in reflexes;

* other conditions, such as fractures, tumors, and infection.

Imaging tests may be considered when your symptoms develop after an injury and nerve damage is suspected, or your medical history suggests conditions that could affect your spine, such as bone disease, tumors, or infection. Treatment depends on whether the damaged disc has resulted in other conditions, such as osteoarthritis, a true herniated disc, or spinal stenosis. Aren't you glad I played baseball? I learned firsthand about back and spine injuries so I take very special care in making the right determination unique just to you.

Spinal Canal Stenosis: Spinal stenosis is a condition that is caused by a narrowing of the space surrounding the spinal cord or the spinal nerves. The spinal cord extends from the brain to the bottom of the spine. Along the spinal cord, the spinal nerves exit the spine and extend to the rest of the body.

Together, the spinal cord and spinal nerves perform two important functions. Nerves pass messages from the body to the brain. The sensations we feel, including pain, pressure, vibration, and other sensations, are detected and passed through these spinal nerves, up the spinal cord, and to our brain.

Nerves also send messages the other direction, from the brain to the body. These messages direct muscle functions, both voluntary and involuntary. These signals help us perform all functions from walking to breathing.

In patients with spinal stenosis, these nerves can become compressed or "scrunched", either within the spinal cord itself, or as the spinal nerves exit the spinal cord. Compression of these nerves leads to the common symptoms experienced by those who have spinal stenosis. When the nerves are compressed, abnormal signals are sent to and from the brain, or sometimes the signals don't get past the area of compression and that's when you may experience pain, numbness or weakness.

Spinal stenosis affects men and women equally, and most often is seen in people over the age of 50. People who have careers that are labor intensive requiring hard physical work are more prone to developing symptoms of spinal stenosis. The most common cause of spinal stenosis is arthritis of the spine, and it is uncommon to find this condition in individuals younger than 30 years old. Spinal stenosis may be caused by a wide variety of conditions, all of which lead to a narrowing of the spinal canal. These conditions may be either acquired or inherited. Spinal stenosis is most often caused from spine arthritis, a process that causes bone spurs in the spine which leads to nerve compression. When spinal stenosis does occur in younger people, it is often related to traumatic injury to the spinal column.

Making the diagnosis of spinal stenosis involves a complete evaluation of the spine. The process always begins with a medical history and physical examination. Imaging studies such as x-ray are often used to determine the extent and location of the nerve compression. X-ray is helpful in looking for causes of spinal stenosis including tumors, traumatic injury, spinal arthritis or inherited abnormalities.

The MRI has become the most frequently used study to diagnose spinal stenosis. The MRI uses magnetic signals instead of x-rays to produce accurate and defined images of the spine. MRIs are helpful because they show more structures, including nerves, discs, and ligaments, than seen on x-rays. MRIs are helpful at showing exactly what is causing pressure on the nerves of the spine.

Sciatica: Sciatica is low back pain combined with a pain through the buttock region and down one leg. The leg pain usually goes past the knee and may go farther to the foot. Sometimes, weakness in the leg muscles occurs with sciatica – and it's all because of one big, long nerve system.

The sciatic nerves are the largest nerves in the body and are actually about the size of your little finger. They come out of the spinal column low in the back and then go behind the hip joint, down the buttock, and down the back of the leg to the foot.

Sciatica is different from other forms of low back pain because while the pain most often begins in the back, it usually travels down one lower extremity as well. This is the type of pain you try everything in the world to get rid of – but can't. The pain is usually described as a "shooting pain", like electricity sent through the body all of a sudden. It can also burn like fire or tingle, much like the feeling when your leg goes to sleep. The pain can range from slightly annoying to totally and completely unbearable. Making matters worse, some people have pain in one part of the leg and numbness in another part of the same leg.

Sciatica is caused by irritation of the sciatic nerve. Usually, there is no specific injury that is related to the onset of sciatica. Occasionally, the pain will suddenly begin after lifting something heavy or moving quickly.

A herniated or bulging disc is the most common cause of sciatica. Spinal stenosis will cause sciatica. As mentioned earlier, as we age, the bone can overgrow and put pressure on the sciatic nerve. Many people with spinal stenosis have sciatica on both sides of the back. Sciatica can also be caused by other effects of aging, such as osteoarthritis and fractures due to osteoporosis. A pinched nerve can also cause this painful condition.

The most common symptom from sciatica is pain. Most people describe a deep, severe pain that starts low on one side of the back and then shoots down the buttock and the leg with certain movements. Sciatica can also cause hip pain. The pain is usually worse with both prolonged sitting and standing. Frequently, the pain is made worse by standing from a low sitting position, such as standing up after sitting on a toilet seat.

In most people, the pain is made worse by sneezing, coughing, laughing, or a hard bowel movement. Bending backward can also make the pain worse. You may also notice a weakness in your leg or foot, along with the pain. The weakness may become so bad you can't move your foot.

Sciatica is a clinical diagnosis. In other words, the doctor will be able to make the diagnosis based on your medical history, a physical examination, and your description of your symptoms. If you have had sciatica for only a brief time and you have no sign of any other diseases, no lab studies or X-ray films may be needed.

If the pain has been present for several weeks, you may get special studies of your back: either computerized tomography or magnetic resonance imaging scans. If you have a history of cancer, HIV infection, IV drug use, or you have been taking steroids over a period a time, I may want to see plain X-ray films of your back or a bone scan. Occasionally, laboratory studies requiring a blood draw may be helpful. A complete blood count may suggest infection, anemia due to certain cancers, or other unusual causes of sciatica.

Other tests results such as elevated sedimentation rate may suggest inflammation somewhere in the body. Urinalysis can suggest a kidney stone, if there is blood in the urine, or infection, if there are bacteria and pus in the urine.

Most of the time, the pain associated with sciatica goes away in days to weeks. Pain can become more chronic in a small number of people, leading to some disability. Sciatica tends to reoccur frequently, sometimes without warning. This is where I come in like a masked crusader. My staff will use every available resource to locate the problem and if possible, fix it. We will also show you how you can live as much of a pain-free life as possible.

Migraine and Chronic Headache: There are many types of headaches which range from those caused by simple stress to those caused by disease already within the body itself. Your eyes can cause headaches. Your sinuses can cause headaches. Your environment can cause headaches. The worse types of headaches are migraine headaches and cluster headaches.

Anyone can experience a headache. Nearly two out of three children will have a headache by age 15. More than 9 in 10 adults will experience a headache sometime in their life.

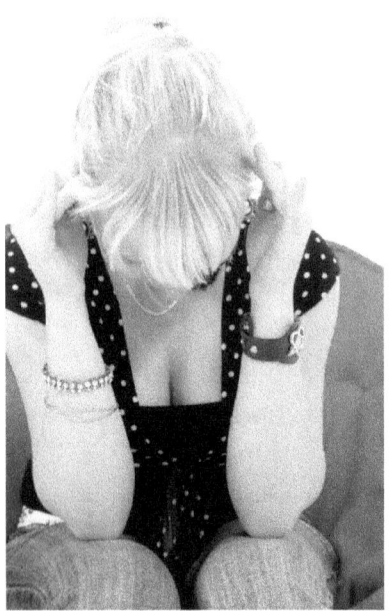

Headache is our most common form of pain and a major reason cited for days missed at work or school as well as visits to the doctor. Without proper treatment, headaches can be severe and interfere with daily activities and worsen.

Certain types of headache run in families. Episodes of headache may ease or even disappear for a time and recur later in life. It's possible to have more than one type of headache at the same time.

Primary headaches occur independently and are not caused by another medical condition. It's uncertain what sets the process of a primary headache in motion. A cascade of events that affect blood vessels and nerves inside and outside the head causes pain signals to be sent to the brain. Brain chemicals called neurotransmitters are involved in creating head pain, as are changes in nerve cell activity.

Migraine, cluster, and tension-type headache are the more familiar types of primary headache.

Secondary headaches are symptoms of another health disorder that causes pain-sensitive nerve endings to be pressed on or pulled or pushed out of place. They may result from underlying conditions including fever, infection, medication overuse, stress or emotional conflict, high blood pressure, psychiatric disorders, head injury or trauma, stroke, tumors, and nerve conditions as described above.

Headaches can range in frequency and severity of pain. Some individuals may experience headaches once or twice a year, while others may experience headaches more than fifteen days a month. Some headaches may recur or last for weeks at a time. Pain can range from mild to disabling and may be accompanied by symptoms such as nausea or increased sensitivity to noise or light, depending on the type of headache.

Headaches as a condition are really very complex. Information about touch, pain, temperature, and vibration in the head and neck is sent to the brain by the trigeminal nerve, a big nerve at the base of the brain. The nerve branches and conducts sensations from the scalp, the blood vessels inside and outside of the skull, the lining around the brain; and the face, mouth, neck, ears, eyes, and throat.

Brain tissue itself lacks pain-sensitive nerves and does not feel pain. Headaches occur when pain-sensitive nerve endings react to headache triggers such as stress, certain foods or odors, or use of medicines and then send messages through the trigeminal nerve to the brain's "relay station" for pain sensation from all over the body. This "relay station" controls the body's sensitivity to light and noise and sends messages to parts of the brain that manage awareness of pain and emotional response to it. Other parts of the brain may also be part of the process, causing nausea, vomiting, diarrhea, trouble concentrating, and other neurological symptoms.

About 12 percent of the U.S. population experience migraines headaches. These headaches are characterized by throbbing and pulsating pain that never lets up and are caused by the activation of nerve fibers that reside within the wall of brain. Blood vessels narrow, temporarily, which decreases the flow of blood and oxygen to the brain. This causes other blood vessels to open wider and increase blood flow.

Migraines involve recurrent attacks of moderate to severe pain that is throbbing or pulsing and often strikes one side of the head. Untreated attacks usually last from four to seventy two hours. Other common symptoms are increased sensitivity to light, noise, and odors; and nausea and vomiting. Routine physical activity, movement, or even coughing or sneezing can worsen the headache pain.

Migraines occur most frequently in the morning, especially upon waking. Some people have migraines at predictable times, such as before menstruation or on weekends following a stressful week of work. Many people feel exhausted or weak following a migraine but are usually symptom-free between attacks.

A number of different factors can increase your risk of having a migraine. These factors, which trigger the headache process, vary from person to person and include sudden changes in weather or environment, too much or not enough sleep, strong odors or fumes, emotion, stress, overexertion, loud or sudden noises, motion sickness, low blood sugar, skipped meals, tobacco, depression, anxiety, head trauma, hangover, some medications, hormonal changes, and bright or flashing lights. Medication overuse or missed doses may also cause headaches. In some fifty percent of migraine sufferers, foods or ingredients can trigger headaches. These include aspartame and other synthetic sweeteners, caffeine – especially caffeine withdrawal, wines and other types of alcohol, chocolate, aged cheeses, food additives, some fruits and nuts, fermented or pickled goods, yeast, and cured or processed meats.

The two major types of migraine are:

The first type is called a migraine with aura, or classic migraine, includes visual disturbances and other neurological symptoms that appear about 10 minutes to an hour before the actual headache and usually last no more than an hour. Individuals may temporarily lose part or all of their vision. The aura may occur without headache pain, which can strike at any time. Other classic symptoms include trouble speaking; an abnormal sensation, numbness, or muscle weakness on one side of the body; a tingling sensation in the hands or face, and confusion. Nausea, loss of appetite, and increased sensitivity to light, sound, or noise may precede the headache.

Migraine without aura, or common migraine, is the more frequent form of migraine. Symptoms include headache pain that occurs without warning and is usually felt on one side of the head, along with nausea, confusion, blurred vision, mood changes, fatigue, and increased sensitivity to light, sound, or noise.

A migraine headache is divided into four phases, all or just some of which may be present during the attack:

The first phase is noticeable symptoms that may occur up to 24 hours prior to developing a migraine. These include food cravings, unexplained mood changes like depression or euphoria, uncontrollable yawning, fluid retention, or increased urination.

The second phase is called aura. Some people will see flashing or bright lights or what looks like heat waves immediately prior to or during the migraine, while others may experience muscle weakness or the sensation of being touched or grabbed.

The third phase is the headache itself. A migraine usually starts gradually and builds in intensity. It is possible to have migraine without a headache.

The final phase is the aftermath. Individuals are often exhausted or confused following a migraine. This period may last up to a full day before you feel healthy and normal again.

Vestibular migraines describe migraine headaches associated with vertigo and are a common cause of balance disorders. We will discuss this a little later in this book.

Migraine treatment is aimed at relieving symptoms and preventing additional attacks. Quick steps to ease symptoms may include napping or resting with eyes closed in a quiet, darkened room; placing a cool cloth or ice pack on the forehead, and drinking lots of fluid, particularly if the migraine is accompanied by vomiting. Small amounts of caffeine may help relieve symptoms during a migraine's early stages.

Everyone who has to live with a migraine needs effective treatment. In general, I believe prevention should be considered if migraines occur one or more times weekly, or if migraines are less frequent yet disabling. Preventive therapy is recommended for individuals who take symptomatic headache treatments of any kind more than three times a week.

Another type of headache, the tension-type headache, is the most common. Its name indicates the role of stress and mental or emotional conflict in triggering the pain and contracting muscles in the neck, face, scalp, and jaw. Tension-type headaches may also be caused by jaw clenching, intense work, missed meals, depression, anxiety, or too little sleep. Sleep apnea may also cause tension-type headaches, especially in the morning. The pain is usually mild to moderate and feels as if constant pressure is being applied to the front of the face or to the head or neck. It also may feel as if a belt is being tightened around the head. Most often the pain is felt on both sides of the head. People who suffer tension-type headaches may also feel overly sensitive to light and sound but there is no pre-headache aura as with migraine. Typically, tension-type headaches usually disappear once the period of stress or related cause has ended.

Tension-type headaches generally affect women slightly more often than men. The headaches usually begin in adolescence and reach peak activity in the thirties. They have not been linked to hormones and do not have a strong hereditary connection.

There are two forms of tension-type headache: Episodic tension-type headaches occur between ten and fifteen days per month, with each attack lasting from thirty minutes to several days. Although the pain is not disabling, the severity of pain typically increases with the frequency of attacks.

Chronic or ongoing tension-type attacks usually occur more than fifteen days per month over a 3-month period. The pain, which can be constant over a period of days or even months, strikes both sides of the head and is more severe and disabling than episodic headache pain. Chronic tension headaches can cause sore scalps and even combing your hair can be painful. Most individuals will have had some form of episodic tension-type headache prior to onset of chronic tension-type headache.

Depression and anxiety can cause chronic tension-type headaches. Headaches may appear in the early morning or evening, when conflicts in the office or at home are anticipated. Other causes include physical postures that strain head and neck muscles such as holding your chin down while reading or holding a phone between your shoulder and ear, degenerative arthritis of the neck, and jaw / joint dysfunctions.

The first step in caring for a tension-type headache involves treating any specific disorder or disease that may be causing it. For example, arthritis of the neck and jaw related joint dysfunction may be helped exercise and corrective devices for the mouth and jaw. Other studies may be needed to detect sleep apnea and should be considered when there is a history of snoring, daytime sleepiness, or obesity.

My training and experience comes in handy in this area. Therapies for chronic tension-type headaches include biofeedback, relaxation training, gentle manipulation, meditation, and cognitive-behavioral therapy to reduce stress. A hot shower or moist heat applied to the back of the neck at just the right time and in just the right way may ease those nightmare symptoms of tension headaches. Many people rely on me and my staff to keep them as headache free as possible by correctly finding the root cause and treating it appropriately the first time around.

Multiple Sclerosis: Multiple sclerosis is a potentially debilitating disease in which your body's immune system eats away at the protective sheath that covers your nerves. This interferes with the communication between your brain and the rest of your body. Ultimately, this may result in deterioration of the nerves themselves, a process that's not reversible.

Symptoms vary widely, depending on the amount of damage and which nerves are affected. People with severe cases of multiple sclerosis may lose the ability to walk or speak. Multiple sclerosis can be difficult to diagnose early in the course of the disease because symptoms often come and go — sometimes disappearing for months.

There's no cure for multiple sclerosis. However treatments can help treat attacks, modify the course of the disease and treat symptoms and ease the pain.

Signs and symptoms of multiple sclerosis vary widely by person, depending on the location of affected nerve fibers. Multiple sclerosis signs and symptoms may include:

- Numbness or weakness in one or more limbs, which typically occurs on one side of your body at a time or the bottom half of your body

- Partial or complete loss of vision, usually in one eye at a time, often with pain during eye movement

- Double vision or blurring of vision

- Tingling or pain in parts of your body

- Electric-shock sensations that occur with certain head movements

- Tremor, lack of coordination or unsteady gait

- Fatigue

- Dizziness

Most people with multiple sclerosis, particularly in the beginning stages of the disease, experience relapses of symptoms, which are followed by periods of complete or partial remission. Signs and symptoms of multiple sclerosis often are triggered or worsened by an increase in body temperature.

The cause of multiple sclerosis is unknown. It's believed to be an autoimmune disease, in which the body's immune system attacks its own tissues. In multiple sclerosis, this process destroys myelin — the fatty substance that coats and protects nerve fibers in the brain and spinal cord.

Myelin can be compared to the insulation on electrical wires. When myelin is damaged, the messages that travel along that nerve may be slowed or even blocked. A combination of factors, ranging from genetics to childhood infections, may play a role.

Factors that may increase your personal risk of developing multiple sclerosis are:

- Being between the ages of 20 and 40. Multiple sclerosis can occur at any age, but most commonly affects people between these ages;

- Being female. Yes, women are about twice as likely as men are to develop multiple sclerosis;

- Having a family history. If one of your parents or siblings has had multiple sclerosis, you have a 1 to 3 percent chance of developing the disease — as compared with the risk in the general population, which is just a tenth of 1 percent. But the experiences of identical twins show that heredity can't be the only factor involved. If multiple sclerosis was determined solely by genetics, identical twins would have identical risks. However, an identical twin has only a 30 percent chance of developing multiple sclerosis if his or her twin already has the disease;

- Having certain infections. A variety of viruses have been linked to multiple sclerosis. Currently the greatest interest is in the association of multiple sclerosis with Epstein-Barr virus, the virus that causes infectious mononucleosis. How Epstein-Barr virus might result in a higher rate of MS remains to be clarified;

- Being white. White people, particularly those whose families originated in northern Europe, are at highest risk of developing multiple sclerosis. People of Asian, African or Native American descent have the lowest risk;

- Living in countries with temperate extremes. Multiple sclerosis is far more common in Europe, southern Canada, northern United States, New Zealand and southeastern Australia. The risk seems to increase with latitude and no one knows why;

- Having certain other autoimmune diseases. You're slightly more likely to develop multiple sclerosis if you have thyroid disease, diabetes or inflammatory bowel disease.

People with multiple sclerosis may also develop muscle stiffness or spasms, paralysis, most typically in the legs, problems with bladder, bowel or sexual function; mental changes, such as forgetfulness or difficulties concentrating, depression, epilepsy and more. Some of the most common types of pain experienced by multiple sclerosis patients include:

*Acute MS pain. This comes on suddenly and may go away just as suddenly. The pain is often intense, but brief in duration. The pain is sometimes referred to as burning, tingling, shooting, or stabbing.

*Trigeminal neuralgia. This is a stabbing pain in the face that can be brought on by almost any facial movement, such as chewing, yawning, sneezing, or washing your face. People with multiple sclerosis typically confuse it with dental pain. Most people can get sudden attacks of pain that can be triggered by touch, chewing, or even brushing the teeth.

*A burning, aching, or a "girdling" feeling around the body. This is called Dysesthesia.

There are also some types of pain related to MS that are described as being chronic in nature -- lasting for more than a month -- including pain from spasticity that can lead to muscle cramps, tight and aching joints, and back or musculoskeletal pain.

Vertigo, Dizziness, Tinnitus and Balance Problems: Balance is defined as a state of equilibrium. It takes significant amount of work for this to occur in the body. The brain uses inputs from many sources to understand where the body is located in relationship to the world around us to allow it to function. Sensory information from the eyes, ears, and position receptors in the rest of the body help keep the body upright and allow it to move in a coordinated fashion. This requires a vast "system" of things which must work in concert with one another – and when one part of the system fails to work properly, the cascade effect will tell you something is wrong by causing vertigo or dizziness. Let's discuss this in depth as I tend to help a lot of patients whose life has been negatively altered by this.

Information located in the base of the brain is transferred from several systems at once; the inner ear, vision from the eyes, and position receptors located throughout the body. They all send signals through the spinal cord. The cerebellum – the part of the brain that uses information to maintain posture, coordinates body motions like walking and fine motor skills, like using a pen to write.

Vertigo, which is a feeling of spinning movement, sometimes accompanied by nausea and vomiting, occurs when any part of that complex system breaks down. However, people tend not to use that word to describe their symptoms but instead use the word dizziness or lightheadedness.

Dizziness is a simple word to say yet is a difficult word to understand and needs to be divided into two categories, either lightheadedness or vertigo. Lightheadedness is the feeling that a person might faint while vertigo is most often described as a spinning sensation with loss of balance. The direction of care is markedly different since lightheadedness may suggest that I investigate things like decreased oxygen or nutrient supply to the brain... due a variety of causes including heart rhythm disturbances or dehydration, while vertigo could send me looking for a neurologic or inner ear cause.

The most important initial step in helping a person with vertigo is to take a through history and understand that you are complaining of spinning symptoms which may be associated with nausea and vomiting and loss of balance among other symptoms.

What is vertigo exactly?

Vertigo is an abnormal sensation that is described as a feeling of spinning or that the world is spinning around them. It is most often associated with an inner ear problem.

The inner ear has two parts, the semicircular canals and the vestibule, which helps the body know where it is in relationship to gravity. There are three semicircular canals which are aligned at right angles to each other and act as the gyroscope for the body. These canals are filled with fluid and are lined with a nerve filled, crystal encrusted membrane that transmits information to the part of the brain that deals with balance and coordination. The cerebellum adds information from sight and from nerve endings in muscles that deal with proprioception, the perception of movement, to help the brain know where it is in relationship to gravity and the world.

Normally, when the head moves, fluid in the semicircular canals shifts and that information is relayed to the brain. When the head stops moving, the fluid stops as well. There may be a slight delay and this is the basis for the vertigo experienced after people participate in many children's games and carnival rides. When a person goes on a merry-go-round or spins quickly around in circles, the fluid in the canals develops momentum and even though the head stops spinning, the fluid may continue to move. This causes vertigo or a spinning sensation and may cause the person to fall or stumble in a crooked line. It also may be associated with vomiting.

In some people with vertigo, inflammation or irritation of the crystals on the nerve membrane that lines the walls of the ear canals may cause the spinning sensation even without much head movement. Often, only one canal is involved and the person may be symptom free if they don't move.

While there are many causes of vertigo, the major distinction is between central causes of vertigo and peripheral causes. Central causes occur because of an abnormality in the cerebellum of the brain.

Distinguishing between central and peripheral causes for disease is an important concept in evaluating neurologic problems. The brain and spinal cord make up the central nervous system while the peripheral nervous system describes the nerves outside the central area. Sometimes it is easy to make the distinction, other times it is more difficult to distinguish between central and peripheral causes. For example, if a person hits their funny bone on your elbow and then develops pain and numbness in their hand, it is mainly due to a direct blow to the ulnar nerve at the elbow. This is a peripheral nerve problem and most people would not seek medical care. If however, a person's leg became numb and weak, the cause may be central - perhaps a stroke in the brain - or there may be a peripheral cause like sciatica or nerve impingement.

Our orientation in space and, therefore, our balance or equilibrium, is primarily measured by three sensory systems:

1. The eye (visual) system

2. The balance (vestibular) system of the inner ear

 3. The general sensory system that transfers information about motion, pressure, and position sensors in joints, muscles, and the skin.

These three systems continuously feed information to the brainstem and the brain about our position in space relative to gravity and the world. The brainstem connects the brain to the spinal cord. The brain, in turn, processes the data and uses the information to make adjustments of our head, body, joints, and eyes. When all three sensory systems and the brain are properly functioning, the final result is a healthy balance system.

Visual input shows the brain where it is in space and time, what direction it is facing, what direction it is moving, and whether it is turning or standing still. Simple tasks like walking and picking up an object are much easier if we can see our surroundings. Feeling seasick is a problem resulting from a miscommunication between a healthy visual system and a healthy inner ear or vestibular system. In this circumstance, the ears are telling the brain that there is movement, while the eyes may be seeing the fixed surroundings of the cabin. Changes in visual acuity, glaucoma, and cataracts are examples of visual problems that in some individuals may be enough to give them a balance disorder.

The inner ear or labyrinth as it's called, is located deep inside in relation to the outer ear and middle ear, and is encased within the temporal bone of the skull. The vestibular structures of the inner ear are the vestibule and three semicircular canals. These structures work together somewhat like a carpenter's level - a tool used to show how "level" a horizontal or vertical surface is - or a gyroscope. Information is sent by way of the vestibulocochlear nerve to the cerebellum of the brain, the part that processes information regarding body balance and position. The rest of the inner ear, the cochlea, is concerned with hearing.

The vestibular system measures linear and rotational movement. A number of disorders can cause this system to stop working or provide inappropriate information. These disorders include everything from pinched nerves to ear infections to tumors to trauma.

The sensory body system that measures motion, position, and pressure via sensors in the skin, muscles, and joints is called the peripheral sensory system. These sensors provide important touch and position information to keep us balanced. For example, if someone pushes you from behind, a slight increase will occur in the activity of the pressure sensors in the balls of the feet. As these sensors note the increased pressure, the brain is notified, and it knows from experience that the body is being pushed forward. The brain then uses this information to tell the body to shift a small amount of weight backward to prevent the body from toppling forward.

The brain processes the information from the three sensory systems. Any problem that interferes with the proper functioning of the central nervous system can lead to a balance problem. Unlike the problems associated with the three sensory input systems discussed above, however, with central nervous system problems, it is unusual to have vertigo as the only symptom. The most common causes of vertigo are peripheral and generally involve the inner ear or labyrinth.

Some of the most common causes of vertigo are:

* Benign paroxysmal positional vertigo. This may be caused when the crystals in the inner ear become dislodged and irritate the semicircular canals. Often the cause is not found but there may be an association with unusual positioning or movement of the head. It is most frequently seen in people older than 60.

* Labyrinthitis, a swelling of the inner ear may follow a viral infection which causes inflammation within the middle ear.

* Meniere's disease, which is a grouping of symptoms associated with vertigo, hearing loss and tinnitus or ringing in the ears which we will discuss in just a minute.

* Acoustic neuroma, which is a benign tumor of the ear that can present with vertigo.

* Inner ear trauma may be due to a variety of mechanisms – even playing football like I did when I was young. A basilar skull fracture may damage the labyrinth system directly or a concussion, where that area of the skull is shaken and may dislodge some of the inner ear crystals causing symptoms of vertigo.

* The inner ear may also be affected by something called barotrauma, a condition where pressure changes may be the causes of damage and vertigo. This type of injury is seen when an individual dives into water and the air in the external ear canal is compressed and damages the ear drum, middle, and inner ear. Barotrauma may also occur as a consequence

of diving where an increase of air pressure within the middle and inner ear can cause structures to rupture. This may cause loss of hearing if the tympanic membrane or ear drum ruptures, or it may cause vertigo if the round and oval windows in the inner ear are damaged.

* Central causes of vertigo that arise in the brain are much less common. Strokes, tumors, seizures, and multiple sclerosis may be associated with vertigo.

* Vestibular migraines describe migraine headaches associated with vertigo and are a common cause of balance disorders. Migraine is a blood vessel or vascular disease which is characterized by periodic, usually one-sided, headaches. These headaches are often preceded for a variable time by associated neurological symptoms, called the aura. Vertigo may occur in individuals with migraine as part of the migraine aura or separately. In younger patients, the vertigo may predate the onset of headaches entirely. A family history of migraine is very common and may be a clue that a balance disorder may be migraine related.

While individuals may use the word dizziness, vertigo symptoms are described by the feeling that either the world is spinning around them or that they themselves are spinning around the world. This is the same type of sensation when a person quickly steps off a merry-go-round or when they twirl themselves and then quickly stops. The feeling of spinning may be associated with loss of balance to the point that the person walks unsteadily or falls down. An onlooker may describe the person walking as if they were drunk.

Vertigo itself is a symptom or indicator of an underlying balance problem, either involving the labyrinth of the inner ear or the cerebellum of the brain. If other structures of the ear are involved, associated symptoms may include decreased hearing and ringing in the ear, called tinnitus.

If there are issues with the cerebellum area of the brain, the person may also complain of difficulty with coordination. Nausea and vomiting are often associated symptoms with vertigo. Frequently, the more intense the vertigo, the more intense the nausea and vomiting become. These symptoms may be so severe that the individual becomes dehydrated and weak and honestly unable to function.

Vertigo is diagnosed by history and physical examination. It is important to confirm the symptom before proceeding to the cause. The key begins with the true understanding the patient's chief complaint and proceeds from there. I may ask questions in regard to what makes the vertigo worse, what makes the spinning better, and whether there are other associated signs including loss of hearing, tinnitus - ringing in the ears, and about any nausea and vomiting. Past medical history and medication use may offer clues as to the cause.

Physical examination is helpful in confirming the presence of nystagmus, which is the abnormal eye motion that the body uses to try to compensate for the abnormal balance signals coming to the brain. A full neurologic exam may be done to make certain that the cause of vertigo is peripheral and due to inner ear issues rather than central problems with the brain. Testing for balance and coordination may help decide if the cerebellum is working properly.

Balance disorders are often unpredictable. Depending on the cause, symptoms may occur at any time, even after long periods without any symptoms. It is important to be cautious in order to avoid accidents that could be caused by a balance disorder.

Carpal Tunnel Syndrome: Last things first – did you notice the name of the condition? The last word of the condition name is "syndrome". A syndrome means that more than just one thing or cause is involved, and that's the case here because it involves the wrist and everything associated with it.

The wrist is surrounded by a band of fibrous tissue that normally functions as a support for the joint. The tight space between this fibrous band and the wrist bone is called the carpal "tunnel" because it is a literal tunnel for this fibrous band. The median nerve passes through the carpal tunnel to receive sensations from the thumb, index, and middle fingers of the hand. Any condition that causes swelling or a change in position of the tissue within the carpal tunnel can squeeze and irritate the median nerve. Irritation of the median nerve in this manner causes tingling and numbness of the thumb, index, and the middle fingers -- a condition known as carpal tunnel syndrome.

People with carpal tunnel syndrome feel numbness and tingling of the hand in the area of the median nerve, which includes the thumb, index, middle, and part of the fourth fingers. These sensations are often more pronounced at night and can awaken people from their sleep. The reason the symptoms are worse at night may be related to the flexed-wrist sleeping position and fluid accumulating around the wrist and hand while hand itself is lying flat. Carpal tunnel syndrome may be a temporary condition that completely resolves or it can persist and progress.

As the condition worsens, you may develop a burning sensation or cramping and weakness of the hand affected. Decreased grip strength can lead to frequent dropping of objects. Occasionally, sharp shooting pains can be felt in the forearm. Chronic carpal tunnel syndrome can also lead to wasting called atrophy of the hand muscles, particularly those near the base of the thumb in the palm of the hand.

The diagnosis of carpal tunnel syndrome is suspected based on the symptoms and the distribution of the hand numbness. Examination of the neck, shoulder, elbow, pulses, and reflexes will be performed to exclude other conditions that can mimic carpal tunnel syndrome. The wrist will be examined for swelling, warmth, tenderness, deformity, and discoloration. Sometimes tapping the front of the wrist can reproduce tingling of the hand, and is referred to as "Tinel's" sign of carpal tunnel syndrome. Symptoms can also at times be reproduced by bending the wrist forward.

The diagnosis is strongly suggested when a nerve conduction velocity test is abnormal. This test involves measuring the rate of speed of electrical impulses as they travel down a nerve. In carpal tunnel syndrome, the impulse slows as it crosses through the carpal tunnel. A test of muscles of the extremity called an electromyogram is sometimes performed to exclude or detect other conditions that might mimic carpal tunnel syndrome, like wrist swelling associated with pregnancy.

Blood tests may be performed to identify medical conditions associated with carpal tunnel syndrome. These tests include thyroid hormone levels, complete blood counts, and blood sugar and protein analysis. X-rays of the wrist and hand might also be helpful to identify abnormalities of the bones and joints of the wrist. We will discuss blood and other tests along with body chemistry a little later in this book.

The choice of treatment for carpal tunnel syndrome depends on the severity of the symptoms and any underlying disease that I might find which could be causing symptoms.

Pregnancy Back Pain: Back pain is one of the most common complained of discomforts during pregnancy. It's like hauling around a ten pound bowling ball tied to your midriff for several months. As your baby grows, your uterus expands to as much as one thousand times its original size. This amount of this type of growth—especially when centered in one specific area—affects the balance of your body and may very easily cause discomfort in the back. This is called pregnancy back pain.

Pregnancy back pain caused by strain on the back muscles usually occurs in mid-pregnancy, when your uterus becomes heavier and your center of gravity changes. Your posture changes in response. Most women begin to lean backward in the later months of pregnancy, which makes their back muscles work harder.

Weakness of the abdominal muscles also can cause back pain. The abdominal muscles normally support the spine and play an important role in the health of the back. During pregnancy, these muscles become stretched and may weaken, causing back pain. These changes also make you more prone to injury when you exercise.

Pregnancy hormones may contribute to back pain. To make your baby's passage through your pelvis easier, a hormone relaxes the ligaments in the strong, weight-bearing joints in the pelvis. This loosening makes the joints more flexible, but it can cause back pain if the joints become too mobile.

Exercises can help lessen that nagging backache. They strengthen and stretch muscles that support the back and legs and promote good posture—keeping the muscles of the back, abdomen, hips, and upper body strong. These exercises not only will help ease back pain but also help prepare you for labor and delivery. Staying active during pregnancy can help with back pain. Water exercise and walking are safe to do during pregnancy and are great for the back too.

Remember, if you have severe pain, or if pain persists for more than 2 weeks, you need to have it evaluated by a qualified healthcare practitioner. Do not try to treat yourself because back pain also can be caused by other problems. Back pain is one of the main symptoms of preterm labor.

Gentle chiropractic manipulation helps realign the shifted vertebra to correct the problem.

Once other causes are ruled out, a maternity girdle may be recommended, a special elastic sling, or back brace. These devices help support the weight of your abdomen and ease the tension on your back. In severe cases, bed rest, or other forms of therapy may be recommended.

These nightmare-like conditions can be helped by using specific metabolic, neurological and physical testing and treatments which I call the testing and treatment triangle!

Testimonial

Patient: Corina J. Sanfino

Chief Complaint Treated: Fibromyalgia Symptoms

Chiropractic care has immensely improved my life! My pain is gone and I can move more easily. When I first went to Dr. Coniglio I was in tears because of my lower back and shoulder pain.

He planned out what care I needed and gave me holistic resolutions which were overall healthier for me as an individual. I have no pain now and can resolve any by alternative means such as exercise, healthy eating and supplemental herbal vitamins.

I felt as though each and every employee in this office cared about each individual who came in for care. I could see it not only in my care, but in the care of others who were there at the same time I was. The plan that Dr. Coniglio made was individualized just for me as well.

I was thrilled with the results of care over the 20-weeks I went here for care. He included adjustments, stim and ice, and a couple of short massages because of the medical condition that was found in my shoulders and lower back.

I would highly recommend this wellness center to friends or family members! Dr. Coniglio is professional, intelligent and came highly recommended to me. He has helped not only me, but many others who struggled through arthritis, car accidents, sports accidents and medical reasons. I found great success using chiropractic care!

Chapter Three

Metabolic Testing and Treatment

I pride myself on performing the most detailed examination possible to best identify the absolute and exact cause of our patient's condition. There are three types of evaluations and testing that we do to identify the patient's problem: Metabolic, neurologic and physical.

Our human body gets the energy we need from food through a process called metabolism, which is the chemical reactions which occur inside the cells of the body that converts the fuel from food into the energy needed to do everything required to maintain and experience life. Specific proteins in the body control the chemical reactions of metabolism, and each chemical reaction is coordinated with other body functions. In fact, thousands of metabolic reactions happen at the same time — all regulated by the body — to keep our cells healthy and working.

Metabolism is a constant process that begins when we're conceived and ends when we die. It is a vital process for all life forms — not just humans. If metabolism stops, you die.

Neurology is the medical application of neuroscience which is the scientific study of the nervous system of the human body. Chiropractic neurology marries the biomechanics and orthopedic aspect of chiropractic care with the latest techniques of assessment and rehabilitation of the central nervous system. The result is a model of diagnosis and care that incorporates all of the patient's symptoms into one complete treatment plan. The result is a treatment that is uniquely specific for your body and your brain. Best of all, this option is natural and non-invasive.

A physical examination with tests, together with a medical history is used to assist in the diagnosis process. Physical examinations are great for the fact that they can be interpreted immediately. Physical examinations are not only reserved for

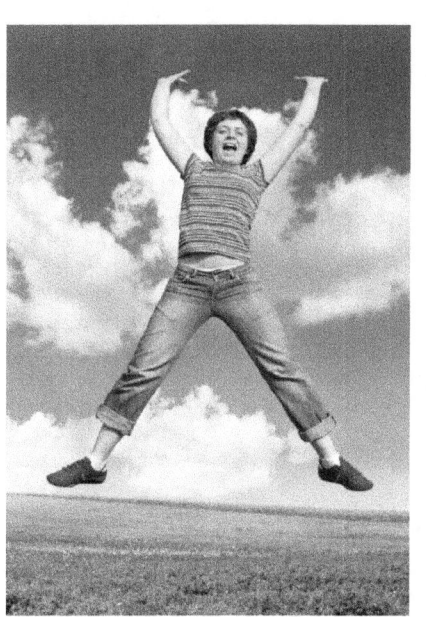

patients experiencing symptoms, but also recommended as a way of ensuring your general health is good – you won't always notice symptoms when something is wrong. For example, your blood pressure may be high but you may not be experiencing any obvious symptoms.

Together, I call this the testing and treatment triangle.

The first side of the triangle deals with your unique body metabolism. In order to see how the chemicals in your body are interacting with other chemicals; known as metabolism – we may do a blood draw, saliva and stool testing. Each chemical in the body has a good value and a bad value. Good values mean that there is just the right amount so that the body works as it should and metabolism is happening without problems. Bad values either in the high or low range, can lead to problems which are sometimes immediate. A good example of this is if a chemical called potassium is low. This low value can affect the way you act, think and even move. Once this low value is brought back to normal again, you will feel like a completely different person because you will be able to function normally again.

Let's take a look at the more common blood tests we scrutinize here at the clinic. We can assess your thyroid, adrenal glands, liver, kidneys, red/white blood cells and gut function with the above lab tests. All internal functions are affected by chronic health conditions. By addressing any problems associated with your thyroid, adrenal glands, your blood chemistry, or gut function we can help you to heal faster. We also check your blood glucose levels since glucose and oxygen are needed by the brain to function properly. By looking over these blood tests and the associated values, we can easily identify any chemicals, nutrients and substances that may be out of alignment. Then, we fix things for you!

The more common blood tests we use are:

- A thyroid panel;

- A complete metabolic panel, called a CMP for short;
- A lipid panel;

- A CBC, which is a complete blood chemistry with auto differential to identify abnormal high or low values.

Thyroid Panel: This tests the body for chemicals which are either produced by your thyroid gland or that affect your thyroid gland function directly. Those chemicals are named TSH, T3 and T4.

TSH is a laboratory test that measures the amount of thyroid stimulating hormone (TSH) in your blood. TSH is produced by the pituitary gland and tells the thyroid gland to make and release the hormones thyroxine (T4) and triiodothyronine (T3). The thyroid gland is a small butterfly shaped organ that lies across your windpipe.

This test is taken to determine if your thyroid gland is working properly. An underactive thyroid gland called hypothyroidism can cause symptoms such as weight gain, tiredness, dry skin, and constipation, a feeling of being too cold or frequent menstrual periods. An overactive thyroid called hyperthyroidism can cause symptoms such as weight loss, rapid heart rate, nervousness, diarrhea, a feeling of being too hot, or irregular menstrual periods.

T3 uptake is a test that measures the level of thyroid hormone-binding proteins in the blood. This test helps estimate the availability of thyroxin binding globulin (TBG), which is the protein that carries most of the T3 and T4 in the blood. The higher the level of TBG, the lower the value of T3 will be. A higher T3 value means less TBG is available, possibly as a result of hyperthyroidism.

T4, or thyroxine, is a hormone produced by the thyroid gland. This test measures the amount of T4 in your blood. This test should be ordered if you have signs of a thyroid disorder. Thyroid function is complex and depends on the action of many different hormones, including thyroid-stimulating hormone and T3. T4 levels are important, because T4 increases numerous substances that produce energy for the body. Most T4 is transported by proteins. If T4 is not attached to a protein, it is called "free" T4.

A comprehensive metabolic panel or CMP is a blood test that provides information about:

- how the kidney and liver are functioning
- sugar (glucose) and protein levels in the blood
- the body's electrolyte and fluid balance

A CMP may be ordered to help diagnose conditions such as diabetes, or liver or kidney disease. The CMP may also be used to monitor chronic conditions, or when a patient is taking medications that can cause certain side effects.

The CMP helps evaluate:

- Glucose, a type of sugar used by the body for energy. Abnormal levels can indicate diabetes and hypoglycemia or low blood sugar.

- Calcium, which plays an important role in muscle contraction, transmitting messages through the nerves, and the release of hormones. Elevated or decreased calcium levels may indicate a hormone imbalance or problems with the kidneys, bones, or pancreas.

- Albumin and total blood protein, which are needed to build and maintain muscles, bones, blood, and organ tissue. The CMP measures albumin specifically, which is the major blood protein produced by the liver, as well as the amount of all proteins in the blood. Low levels may indicate liver or kidney disease or nutritional problems.

- Sodium, potassium, carbon dioxide, and chloride (electrolytes), which help regulate the body's fluid levels and its acid-base balance. They also play a role in regulating heart rhythm, muscle contraction, and brain function. Abnormal levels also may occur with heart disease, kidney disease, or dehydration.

- Blood urea nitrogen (BUN) and creatinine, which are waste products filtered out of the blood by the kidneys. Increased concentrations in the blood may signal a decrease in kidney function.

- Alkaline phosphatase (ALP), alanine amino transferase (ALT), aspartate amino transferase (AST), and bilirubin; ALP, ALT, and AST are liver enzymes; bilirubin is produced by the liver. Elevated concentrations may indicate liver dysfunction.

The CMP is more accurate when performed after fasting, so you may be asked not eat for 8 to 12 hours before the test.

A Lipid Panel: Lipid is just a medically fancy word which means fat. This is another name for a complete cholesterol test — also called a lipid panel or lipid profile and is a blood test that can measure the amount of cholesterol and triglycerides in your blood. A cholesterol test can help determine your risk of atherosclerosis, the buildup of plaques in your arteries that can lead to narrowed or blocked arteries throughout your body which may lead to a heart attack or a stroke. High cholesterol levels usually don't cause signs or symptoms, so a cholesterol test is an important tool. High cholesterol levels are a significant risk factor for heart disease.

When we take blood for a lipid panel we measure four types of fats in your blood for their good verses bad values:

- Total cholesterol. This is a sum of your blood's cholesterol content.

- High-density lipoprotein (HDL) cholesterol. This is sometimes called the "good" cholesterol because it helps carry away LDL cholesterol, thus keeping arteries open and your blood flowing more freely.

- Low-density lipoprotein (LDL) cholesterol. This is sometimes called the "bad" cholesterol. Too much of it in your blood causes the buildup of fatty deposits in your arteries which reduces blood flow. These deposits sometimes rupture and can lead to a heart attack or stroke.

- Triglycerides. Triglycerides are a specific type of fat in the blood. When you eat, your body converts any calories it doesn't need into triglycerides, which are stored in fat cells. High triglyceride levels usually mean you regularly eat more calories than you burn. High levels are also seen in overweight people, in those who eat too many sweets or drink too much alcohol, and in people with diabetes who have elevated blood sugar levels.

Cholesterol testing is very important if you:

- Have a family history of high cholesterol or heart disease

- Are overweight

- Are physically inactive

- Have diabetes

- Eat a high-fat diet

These factors put you at increased risk of developing high cholesterol and heart disease. Don't forget that cholesterol is often high during pregnancy, so pregnant women should keep on top of this when visiting us for relief of back pain.

CBC with Auto Diff: This is medical shorthand for the Complete Blood Count and Automated Differential Count. The CBC is really a series of lab tests that measure the amount, shapes, and sizes of red and white blood cells in a sample of your blood. The CBC is also used to diagnose various illnesses. The differential count measures the different types of white blood cells and compares their amounts to the total count in the volume. The CBC measures:

Red Blood Cells or RBCs

Several tests that measure the status of RBCs are included in the CBC. The RBC measures the number of red blood cells in one cubic millimeter of blood. Hematocrit measures the percentage of total blood volume that consists of RBCs. The results of these lab tests give a good picture of the health of the RBCs and their ability to carry oxygen and nutrients throughout your body.

White Blood Cells or WBCs

The WBC count has two parts. The first is a total count, which measures the number of WBCs in one cubic millimeter of blood. The second is the differential count, which measures the number and percentage of each type of WBCs present in the specimen. Increases and decreases in any of these numbers can be used to diagnose many common conditions because white blood cells are produced in response to infection.

Platelet Count

The platelet count is a measure of the number of platelets per cubic millimeter of blood. Platelets are involved in clotting of the blood.

Blood Smear

A blood smear is the microscopic examination of a sample of the blood. Counts of RBCs and WBCs are performed, and looked at carefully for variations in size and shape among the visible cells.

Sensitivity Testing: This test determines if you have sensitivity to gluten found in wheat, rye, barley and milk, eggs, yeast, and soy. If you are sensitive to any of these food groups, you can take it to the bank that it's making your condition worse! If you have any of the following symptoms, you could be suffering from sensitivity to gluten, soy, milk, eggs or yeast:

- Suffering from chronic pain or fatigue

- Suffering from frequent indigestion

- Suffering from bloating after eating

- Suffering from frequent loose bowel movements

- Experience constipation regularly

- Suffering from mouth ulcers or sores

- If you regurgitate partially or throw up often

The term we have all heard for years, "You are what you eat," has more truth than meets the eye. There are general healthy eating guidelines for everyone, but many times the recommended foods will not make everyone feel and look healthy. Only 2% of Americans suffer from true clinically diagnosed food allergies, however, many suffer from undiagnosed food sensitivities or intolerances. It is estimated that 5% of food allergies are immediate and 95% are delayed. Delayed food reactions are known as cyclic. The recurrent ingestion of the offending food such as milk or wheat can mask the symptoms, go unrecognized and are delayed with no cause and effect relationship.

A few common but little known unsuspected symptoms or conditions that may be related to food allergy or sensitivity are:

- GI symptoms - gas, belching, fatigue after meals, intermittent diarrhea, and constipation

- Spastic Colon

- Irritable bowel syndrome

- Skin rashes

- Itchy eyelids

- Vertigo

- Tinnitus (with normal hearing and other causes ruled out)

- Post nasal drip

- Asthma or asthma bronchitis
Sinus or migraine headaches

Food allergies and sensitivities are broad in definition, classification, variety, number and intensity of symptoms and associated medical conditions.

The only way to find out if you are suffering from any of these sensitivities is to run the test!

Adrenal Stress Index or ASI: We can further test your adrenal glands with a test called an Adrenal Stress Index. This is a salivary test much like DNA testing. Your adrenal glands are your "stress" organs meaning that they react to stress. If you have been or are currently under stress, this test is a must!

If you have problems going to sleep or staying asleep, or controlling your blood sugar, we will check cortisol levels. When your body's cortisol levels are abnormal, you will suffer from insomnia and/or problems with your blood sugar. Cortisol levels can be corrected via specific nutritional guidance.

The Immune System: The immune system is made up of special cells, proteins, tissues, and organs and defends your body against germs and microorganisms we come in contact with every day. In most cases, the immune system does a great job of keeping people healthy and preventing infections. But sometimes problems with the immune system can lead to illness and infection. Through a series of steps called "immune response", the immune system attacks organisms and substances that invade the body and cause disease.

The immune system is made up of a vast network of cells, tissues, and organs that all work together to protect the body. The cells involved are white blood cells, or leukocytes, which come in two basic types that combine to seek out and destroy disease-causing organisms or substances.

Leukocytes are produced or stored in many locations in the body, including the thymus, spleen, and bone marrow. For this reason, they're called the lymphoid organs. There are also clumps of lymphoid tissue throughout the body, primarily as lymph nodes, that house and store the leukocytes.

The white blood cells circulate through the body between the organs and nodes via lymphatic vessels and blood vessels. In this way, the immune system works in a coordinated manner to monitor the body for germs or substances that might cause problems.

The two basic types of white blood cells are:

- Phagocytes, cells that literally chew up invading germs, and;

- Lymphocytes, cells that allow the body to remember and recognize previous invaders and help the body destroy them.

63

When foreign substances that invade the body are detected, several types of cells work together to recognize them and respond much like an EMT would do to an accident. These cells trigger antibodies, specialized proteins that lock onto specific antigens. Once produced, these antibodies continue to exist in a person's body, so that if the same antigen is presented to the immune system again, the antibodies are already there to do their job. So if someone gets sick with a certain disease, like chickenpox, that person typically doesn't get sick from it again. That is why a blood test called immune panels is so important.

There are two parts to the immune system and they are called TH1 and TH2. TH1 cells are called T-cells or T-Helper cells. T-cells are like the armed forced of the human body that attack and cleans up after a sickness.TH2 cells are also called B-cells. B-cells produce the antibodies which our bodies use to fight off germs and viruses. They tell T-cells what to kill, like the commander of the armed forces would do.

In autoimmune disorders, the immune system mistakenly attacks the body's healthy organs and tissues as though they were foreign invaders. Autoimmune diseases include:

- Lupus, a chronic disease marked by muscle and joint pain and inflammation and is the abnormal immune response also may involve attacks on the kidneys and other organs;

- Rheumatoid arthritis, a disease in which the body's immune system acts as though certain body parts such as the joints of the knee, hand, and foot are foreign tissue and attacks them;

- Scleroderma, a chronic autoimmune disease that can lead to inflammation and damage of the skin, joints, and internal organs;

- Ankylosing spondylitis, a disease that involves inflammation of the spine and joints, causing stiffness and pain, and;

- Dermatomyositis, a disorder marked by inflammation and damage of the skin and muscles.

Allergic disorders occur when the immune system overreacts to exposure to triggers in the environment. The substances that provoke such attacks are called allergens. The immune response can cause symptoms such as swelling, watery eyes, sneezing and even a life-threatening reaction called anaphylaxis. Allergic disorders include:

Asthma, a respiratory disorder that can cause breathing problems and frequently involves an allergic response by the lungs. If the lungs are oversensitive to certain allergens like pollen, molds, animal dander, or dust mites, it can trigger breathing tubes in the lungs to become narrowed, leading to reduced airflow and making it hard for a person to breathe. Eczema is an itchy rash also known as atopic dermatitis. Although this is not necessarily caused by an allergic reaction, it more often occurs in kids and teens who have allergies, hay fever, or asthma or who have a family history of these conditions.

Other allergies include environmental allergies to dust mites, for example, seasonal allergies such as hay fever, drug allergies which are reactions to specific medications or drugs, food allergies such as to nuts and allergies to toxins like bee stings are the common conditions people usually refer to as allergies.

Immune Panels: As you know, an autoimmune disorder is when your immune system attacks a particular area of the body such as your nervous system, joints, connective tissue, thyroid and more. We test for specific antibodies to determine if you suffer from an autoimmune condition. The immune panels give me an in depth picture as to what is exactly happening with your immune system. If you are suffering from an auto-immune disorder, it obviously trumps everything and it must be the first thing to be addressed. Some examples are:

- Rheumatoid Arthritis affecting your joints

- Sjogren's Syndrome affecting the moisture producing glands

- Scleroderma affecting the connective tissue

- Hashimoto's affecting the thyroid

- Grave's Disease affecting the thyroid

- Multiple Sclerosis affecting the brain and spinal cord

- Celiac Disease affecting the intestinal tract

- Addison's Disease affecting the adrenal gland

- Pernicious Anemia affecting the body cells

- Myasthenia Gravis affecting the muscles

- Dermatomyositis affecting the skin and muscles

- Reynaud's Disease affecting the extremities

- Type 1 Diabetes affecting the pancreatic function

H.Pylori: H. pylori is a common infection of the stomach. It may actually be the most common infection in the world. It is now clear that the infection is directly related to the development of stomach and duodenal ulcers, and it is very likely that it may be related to cancers involving the stomach.

When food is swallowed, it passes through the esophagus, the tube that connects the throat to the stomach. It then enters the larger upper part of the stomach. A strong acid that helps to break down the food is secreted in the stomach. The narrower, lower part of the stomach is called the antrum. The antrum contracts frequently and vigorously, grinding up the food and squirting it into the small intestine. The duodenum is the first part of the small intestine, just beyond the stomach. The stomach, including the antrum, is covered by a layer of mucous that protects it from the strong stomach acid.

It is known that alcohol, aspirin, and arthritis drugs such as ibuprofen can interrupt the protective mucous layer. This allows the strong stomach acid to injure underlying stomach cells. In some people, drugs, smoking and stress appear to contribute in some way.

H. pylori is really a fragile type of bacteria that seems to find an ideal home in the protective mucous layer of the stomach. These bacteria by shape have long threads protruding from them that attach to the underlying stomach cells. The mucous layer that protects the stomach cells from acid also protects H. pylori. These bacteria do not actually invade the stomach cells as certain other bacteria can. The infection, however, is very real and it does cause the body to react – sometimes in really strange ways. As infection-fighting white blood cells move into the area the body develops H. pylori antibodies in the blood.

H. pylori infection probably occurs when an individual swallows the bacteria in food, fluid, or perhaps from contaminated utensils. The infection is likely one of the most common worldwide. The rate of infection increases with age, so it occurs more often in older people. It also occurs frequently in young people in the developing countries of the world, since the infection tends to be more common where sanitation is poor or living quarters are cramped. In many cases it does not produce symptoms. In other words, the infection can occur without the person knowing it. The infection remains localized to the gastric area, and persists unless specific treatment is initiated.

Intestinal Permeability: The lining of the intestines is a barrier that normally only allows properly digested fats, proteins, and starches to pass through and enter the bloodstream. It allows substances to pass in several ways. Chloride, potassium, magnesium, sodium and free fatty acids cross through intestinal cells. Proteins, fatty acids, glucose, minerals, and vitamins also cross through cells, but they do it by different way.

There's a third way substances can pass through which involve spaces in between the cells that line the intestines. These tight junctions are called "desmosomes". When the intestinal lining becomes irritated, the junctions loosen and allow unwanted larger molecules in the intestines to pass through into the blood. These unwanted substances are seen by the immune system as foreign because they aren't normally present in blood. This triggers an antibody reaction.

When the intestinal lining becomes further damaged, even larger substances, such as disease-causing bacteria, undigested food particles, and toxins, pass directly through these damaged cells. Again, the immune system is alarmed and antibodies and substances called "cytokines" are released. Cytokines alert white blood cells to attack the particles. This fight produces oxidants, which cause irritation and inflammation throughout the body.

Symptoms include abdominal pain, asthma, chronic joint pain, chronic muscle pain, confusion, fuzzy or foggy thinking, gas and indigestion. More serious symptoms can include mood swings, nervousness, poor immunity, recurrent vaginal infections, skin rashes, diarrhea, recurrent bladder infections, poor memory, and shortness of breath, constipation, bloating, aggressive behavior, anxiety and severe fatigue.

Neurotransmitters: In general, the endocrine system, the body system that produces hormones, is in charge of body processes that happen slowly, such as cell growth. Faster processes like breathing and body movement are controlled by the nervous system. But even though the nervous system and endocrine system are separate systems, they often work together to help the body function properly.

The foundations of the endocrine system are the hormones and glands. Hormones are chemical substances that act like messenger molecules in the body. After being made in one part of the body, they travel to other parts of the body where they help control how cells and organs do their work. As the body's chemical messengers, hormones transfer information and instructions from one set of cells to another. Many different hormones move through the bloodstream, but each type of hormone is designed to affect only certain cells. Some carry electrical impulses. These are called neurotransmitters.

We test for decreased brain neurotransmitters.

Neurotransmitters are vital for proper brain function, clarity of thought and more. Decreased levels of neurotransmitters can cause increased pain sensations as well. Like a fast-moving relay race, neurotransmitters, which are actually hormones, are the vehicle by which messages travel from one nerve cell to another in the brain. They affect mood, memory and our ability to concentrate, as well as several physical processes. When these chemical messengers are disrupted, the message may go right back to the transmitter or be lost altogether. When considering mental illness, the result of interrupted neurotransmitters can be depression or even a tendency toward drug and alcohol dependency.

Though the brain has billions of nerve cells, they don't actually touch – thus the job of neurotransmitters is to bring messages back and forth. Because neurotransmitters can impact a specific area of the brain, including behavior or mood, their malfunctions can cause effects ranging from mood swings to aggression and anxiety.

Normally, nerve impulses move along the brain through axons, long cellular structures which act as a roadway for the impulse – until they land at a presynaptic membrane, or a dead end. These membranes house the neurotransmitters that will be sent out into free spaces, or synaptic clefts, so that they can be collected by receptors of another neuron. The neuron that collects the neurotransmitter then internalizes it and the nerve impulse can keep moving forward with the message. If serotonin or norepinephrine movement is interrupted, depression or anxiety can be the result, as these hormones regulate things like mood, appetite and concentration.

Dopamine is another neurotransmitter. Low levels of dopamine may cause schizophrenia, characterized in part by emotional disturbances, but certain medications can help reduce the symptoms. Attention-deficit - hyperactivity disorder or ADHD is also believed to be a result of interrupted passages of dopamine or norepinephrine. Tiredness, high levels of stress and poor motivation are also linked to low dopamine.

Mental illnesses, such as personality disorders and social disorders, are believed to be caused by the interrupted transfer of neurotransmitter messages. Those who suffer with drug or alcohol addictions, the gamma-aminobutyric acid, or GABA, receptor may be affected. This neurotransmitter slows the speed of nerve impulses and causes muscles to relax.

Interestingly, people with vitamin deficiencies may be more likely to experience disrupted, lacking or ineffective neurotransmitters. Amino acids are the building blocks of neurotransmitter production, but amino acids – the building blocks of life, can't be generated without first taking in a broad range of vitamins and minerals. Diets that are too low in protein may also contribute to impaired neurotransmitter function.

Hormone Panels: We can check hormone panels to determine if the males suffer from low testosterone or females suffer from low estrogen/progesterone levels. Symptoms related to decreased hormone levels may include depression, fatigue, mental fogginess, mood swings, hot flashes, sweating attacks, weight gain, and decreased physical stamina.

Traditionally, age-related male hormone changes were not considered challenging because fertility in men persists until an advanced age. Careful evaluation in males shows progressive age-related changes including:

- Decreased muscle mass & strength

- Hair loss

- Decreased vigor, low energy

- Insomnia

- Decreased libido

- Nervousness & Depression

These changes usually begin in the fourth and fifth decades and point towards hormone imbalances and deficiencies which may be considered the male equivalent of menopause, called Andropause.

In females, the hormones we are most concerned about are estrogen, progesterone, and testosterone. These are made in a woman's ovaries, the small almond-shaped sex glands in the pelvis that also produce a woman's eggs. Thought of as the primary female hormone, estrogen builds up the uterine lining, stimulates breast tissue, and thickens the vaginal wall. It also affects almost every other organ in the body. Estrogen plays a critical role in bone building and is thought to have important protective effects on the cardiovascular system.

Progesterone, which is made only during the second half of the menstrual cycle, prepares the uterine lining for an egg to implant, but progesterone also has other important effects on many of the tissues sensitive to estrogen. Testosterone, also made in the ovaries, plays a role in stimulating sexual desire, generating energy, and developing muscle mass.

The balance of hormones in your body at any given point is affected by many factors. The pituitary gland, at the base of your brain, and your ovaries are constantly communicating via their respective hormones, dictating the changing hormone levels of your monthly cycle and the production of eggs. The pituitary produces follicle-stimulating hormone and other hormones. Stress, body weight, time of day, time of the month, and any medications you take can all cause temporary changes in your hormone levels.

Menopause brings major, permanent changes to the hormone levels and hormone balance of your body. The ovaries stop producing eggs, and they also quit producing their hormones. This does not happen all at once. By their late 30s, many women produce less progesterone, which can lead to heavier, more frequent periods early in the "perimenopause" process. Then the ovaries' estrogen production tapers off. It is the fluctuations in estrogen production and, later, the lack of estrogen that primarily brings on the discomforts and health concerns that are associated with menopause.

Fluctuating and falling estrogen levels disrupt your internal thermostat, causing vasomotor instability, the scientific name for the process that causes hot flashes. Your sleep cycles and some muscle tone, most notably in the pelvic area, are also affected by the drastic reduction in estrogen levels.

We can address the problems associated with male and female hormone level imbalances and in many cases take steps to assure decisive positive outcomes to relieve the pain and other associated symptoms.

Inflammation: Many patients suffering from chronic health conditions also suffer from inflammatory processes. Just about every fibromyalgia patient that I have ever treated suffers from some form of chronic inflammatory process throughout their body.

Inflammation is the body's response to cellular injury and without this process, our bodies could not survive. Inflammation represents a protective response designed to rid the body of the initial cause of injury and the consequences of that injury, specific to the cells within the body. Cell injury may occur due to trauma, genetic defects, physical and chemical agents, tissue death, foreign bodies, immune reactions and infections.

Inflammation is a local reactive change that involves the release of antibacterial agents from nearby cells that defend the host against infection. It also facilitates early tissue healing and repair. It contains or "walls off" the infectious or injurious agent and serves as a defense mechanism that the body can use to restore itself to a normal form and function.

There are two types of inflammation: acute and chronic. Acute inflammation is characterized by a rapid onset and short duration. It manifests with an outpouring of fluid and plasma proteins, and emigration of leukocytes, the white cells of the body. Chronic inflammation is of prolonged duration and manifests by the presence of lymphocytes and macrophages or cells that eat bacteria, and results in fibrosis and tissue death. When inflammation continues for prolonged periods of time, it can be thought of as the healing process in overdrive, and changes can occur to localized tissues as well as the entire body.

C-reactive protein, also known as CRP is produced by the liver. The level of CRP rises when there is inflammation throughout the body. The CRP test is a general test to check for inflammation in the body. That means, it can reveal that you have inflammation somewhere in your body, but it cannot pinpoint the exact location.

We may order this test to:

- Check for flare-ups of inflammatory diseases such as rheumatoid arthritis, lupus, or vasculitis

- Determine if anti-inflammatory nutrition is working to treat a disease or condition

A positive test means you have inflammation in the body. This may be due to a variety of different conditions, including:

- Inflammatory bowel disease

- Cancer

- Rheumatic fever

- Tuberculosis

- Heart attack

- Infection

- Connective tissue disease

- Lupus

- Pneumococcal pneumonia

- Rheumatoid arthritis

Glutathione Treatment: We use glutathione in our treatment of all chronic conditions along with nutritional guidance, suggestions and counseling. Glutathione is the "mother-load" of all anti-oxidants. We have seen miraculous changes in our patient population as a result of our specific glutathione protocols.

Glutathione is an essential component of your cells, with low glutathione levels; cells cannot perform many of their functions properly. Although glutathione functions in dozens of roles in our metabolism, the major functions can be summarized in four areas:

*It is the major antioxidant produced by the body. Antioxidants such as vitamins C or E cannot be made by your body and in fact could not work properly if glutathione were not present.

Our immune system depends on a steady supply of glutathione. Without it, our immune defenses become weakened.

*It is important in detoxifying many substances including heavy metals, the breakdown products of cigarettes and automobile exhaust, many cancer-causing agents, and a multitude of pollutants and toxins we encounter on a daily basis.

*The major source of energy produced in our cells is derived from tiny structures called mitochondria – the literal engine of the human cell. These mitochondria would literally burn up without the presence of glutathione.

You might have come across the term "free radicals" before. If you haven't, free radicals are molecules that occur naturally within our bodies. But although they occur naturally they pose a damaging effect to the body. The effects of glutathione as the body's defender are unparalleled. Glutathione in essence is a protein that is produced naturally within each cell when certain components within the body are combined. It acts as the master defender against harmful toxins. Our levels of glutathione are depleted at an accelerated rate when there is an increase in toxins within the body, and the body's ability to produce glutathione decreases incrementally as we age.

*We use glutathione in our treatment of just about all chronic conditions we come across along with nutritional guidance, suggestions and counseling, because it works. Specific dosage and application is important for proper absorption. Please see a qualified physician for proper dosage.

These tests, together with other modalities help me to pinpoint the exact nature of the problem.

Testimonial

Patient: Evelyn Fox

Chief Complaint Treated: Excruciating Migraine Headaches

Chiropractic care has improved my life tremendously! For years I had suffered with really bad headaches, only later to find out they were the worst kind of imaginable migraines. I was prescribed and had taken all kinds of medicines to treat them and although they did go away for a while, they always returned.

One day I was reading an article on migraines and how chiropractic care could help. My family had been going to Coniglio Chiropractic and advised me to schedule an appointment. I kept putting it off for the longest time, then one day after being confined to my room in total darkness I decided to make the call. It was the best decision I ever made!

Since my initial consultation and subsequent visits, I no longer need medication and have not suffered a migraine in almost a year! I still go once a month for my chiropractic care and all I can say is I feel like a new woman!

I would tell a friend or a family member who was curious to give it a try and not to believe everything they hear or read about visiting a chiropractor. It has really helped me and has given me back my life.

What has pleased me the most in the course of my treatment is that has worked! I think Dr. Coniglio and his staff are AWESOME! You are always greeted with a smile and that's so refreshing!

Chapter Four

Neurologic Testing and Treatment

The human nervous system is an intricate and complex network of fibers that flows through the entire body and functions in complicated and often mysterious ways. Sophisticated imaging and laboratory tests do not always provide sufficient information about how the nerves are functioning -- or not functioning, as the case may be. The neurological examination I perform is a series of questions and tests that provide crucial information about the nervous system and how it is functioning. It is an inexpensive, noninvasive way to determine what might be wrong.

The focus and thoroughness of the neurological examination must be tailored to the chief complaint and symptoms by the patient. Here we will detail ways and means which I use to discover the exact nature of that cause and effect relationship between pain and disease process. These tests are designed to examine a wide variety of cognitive abilities, including speed of information processing, attention, memory, language, and executive functions and basic body functions which are necessary for what we call goal-directed behavior. By testing a vast range of cognitive abilities and examining patterns of performance in different areas, I can identify underlying abnormal processes and functions within the body.

The upper brainstem is called the "mesencephalon", the middle and lower parts work together and are known as the "ponto- medullary" region of the brain.

Besides controlling many automatic body processes, the brainstem has a profound effect on our sensitivity to pain and sleep/wake cycles. If our brainstem doesn't function well, neither do these processes – including our blood pressure. We all know that the cerebellum controls balance and coordination but in addition, it sends messages up to the opposite cerebral hemisphere to keep the upper brainstem from over-firing. This is part of a feedback loop in which input goes from the cerebellum to the opposite side of the brain and then back down to the lower brainstem. So, what can go wrong? A lack of firing from the cerebrum down to the lower brainstem results in an inability to perform its duty.

Trauma, emotional, physical and chemical stress can disrupt the normal feedback loop. When the brainstem over-fires a wide range of symptoms may result. Migraine headaches as discussed earlier can be a direct cause of blood vessel dilation due to an over-stimulated brainstem. Fibromyalgia, irritable bowel syndrome, high blood pressure and vertigo are other common symptoms associated with an overactive upper brainstem. Sleep disorders are also related to a high upper brainstem output.

On the other hand, this scenario becomes disrupted as a result of everyday stressors. The way in which this mechanism causes the chronic pain seen in fibromyalgia is simple; an overactive upper brainstem causes the adrenal medulla to release high levels catecholamines and norepinephrine into the blood. Pain receptors become stimulated resulting in intractable pain. For example, your shoulder may hurt one day and the next day the pain has moved to the knee. Pain keeps our blood pressure high, as can kidney problems.

Neurologic Specific Tests

Blood Pressure: Blood pressure is taken on both sides of the body. Normal blood pressure is approximately 120/80. If one side measures higher than the other side, this may indicate decreased brain function. Think of it this way: When you get angry, your blood pressure rises. There is a reason for that. It's your brain telling your body something is wrong.

Oxygen Saturation: The measurement is taken on both sides of the upper extremities with a device called a pulse-oximeter. This is a device to see if the oxygen is properly reaching to the tips of the body in a balanced manner and if so, at what saturation level. Oxygen is carried in the blood attached to hemoglobin or "red" molecules. Oxygen saturation is a measure of how much oxygen the blood is carrying as a percentage of the maximum it could carry. When there is an imbalance we of course go further into the neurological exam to see if the hemispheres are balanced right versus left.

We combine this test with future treatments and we take pre-and-post oxygen saturation levels to see if our neurological treatment is balancing the systemic affects of oxygen.

Computerized Spinal Nerve Testing: A computerized spinal nerve scan is a non-invasive test that enables us to determine abnormal function in the spine, where it is located and exactly what may be wrong.   These tests will give us a visual snapshot of trouble areas in your body, and how improper nerve function may be contributing to specific health conditions you may have. Our standard test is something called spinal thermography, which measures skin temperature differences and nerve energy along the spine and surrounding area.

Since muscles are controlled by nerves, misalignments prevent the nerve from functioning properly. Misalignments can trigger an abnormal flow of electrical current to the muscles. Muscle balance symmetry disassociation occurs when nerve function is impaired by a misalignment, so it creates a muscle imbalance. The surrounding muscles can become weaker or stronger, tighter, or fatigued. The scan reveals a misaligned or unequal muscle pattern and increased tension on one side compared to the other.

Temperature differences along the spine can be seen on a thermal scan. If your body temperature is a normal 98.6 degrees, then both sides of your spine should also be the same temperature. Since the skin is the largest organ of the body, the blood vessels under the skin expand to release heat and contract to retain heat in order to regulate body temperature.

Muscle Stretch Reflexes: The nervous system is very complex network of all body systems working together in harmony, and that includes your muscles. For most major actions in the body the brain must decide what movement or action must be taken, the nerve impulses must be transmitted out of the brain, down the spinal cord and out to the intended receiver. Then when the action is carried out the impulse must return back via the reverse pathway to tell the brain it was completed and start the next process. This is the path for any brain-controlled, conscious, impulses. Although it takes a lot of words to explain, it is really a very rapid process that only takes about a quarter of the time it takes to blink your eye.

There are many processes in the body that do not require direct thought to complete. The heart functions, breathing, metabolic processes, disease fighting and many other autonomic or "automatic" processes happen "automatically" in the body. The body uses signals to increase, decrease, or maintain many of these actions. If the carbon dioxide levels in the body begin to raise, the autonomic nervous system, through acid verses base thermostats, calls for an increase in respiratory rate to compensate.

Another automatic response by the nervous system is the reflex. The body reacts in a predetermined way based on specific stimulus. If you touch something hot and it burns you, then you automatically pull away from the heat. The stretch reflex also known as myotatic reflex is one of those responses.

The stretch reflex; which is also often called the knee-jerk reflex, or deep tendon reflex, is a preprogrammed response by the body to a stretch stimulus in the muscle. When a muscle is stretched an impulse is immediately sent to the spinal cord and a response to contract the muscle is received. Since the impulse only has to go to the spinal cord and back, not all the way to the brain, it is a very quick impulse and therefore happens too quickly for us to control. This is designed as a protective measure for the muscles, to prevent tearing as I did when I played baseball. The muscle is stretched and the impulse is also immediately received to contract the muscle, hopefully protecting it from being pulled forcefully or beyond a normal range.

The "action" or synergistic muscles; those muscles that produce the same movement together to accomplish a specific task, are involved and activated when the stretch reflex is put in motion. This further strengthens the contraction and prevents injury. At the same time, the stretch reflex has an inhibitory aspect to the opposite muscles.

The stretch reflex is very important in posture. It helps maintain proper posturing because a slight lean to either side causes a stretch in the spinal, hip and leg muscles to the other side, which is quickly countered by the stretch reflex. This is a constant process of adjusting and maintaining. The body is constantly under push verses pull force from the outside, one of which is the natural force of gravity.

Another example of the stretch reflex is the knee-jerk test. When the knee tendon is tapped with a small hammer or other device, it causes a slight stretch in the tendon, and consequently the quadriceps muscles. The result is a quick, although mild, contraction of the quadriceps muscles, resulting in a small kicking motion. Any abrupt, forceful stretch on the muscle causes the stretch reflex to fire, in a healthy person. Delays in or absence of the stretch reflex are signs of possible neurological or neuromuscular damage. Many times I can either repair that damage or at minimum, help you cope by presenting alternatives.

Vibratory Sensation: Vibration tests the back part of the spinal cord, known as the dorsal column. Many people think of the spinal cord as a single entity. It is in fact a bundle of connecting nerves, surrounded by several tough layers of material which are designed to protect it from harm. The spinal cord carries signals to and from the brain, which literally requires a lot of wiring to communicate with various parts of the body. The dorsal column is a part of the spinal cord which is responsible for transporting sensory input from the body to the cerebral cortex. This part of the spinal cord is a key player in perceiving fine touch, such as that used to distinguish textures, along with vibration. The dorsal column also contributes to the body's system, used to orient the body in space and to coordinate muscle movements, given information about the body's position.

Damage to the dorsal column causes loss of sensation below the area of damage. Damage can occur as a result of lesions which appear in the case of some diseases and attack the central nervous system, and it may also be caused by trauma such as damage to the spine incurred in a car accident, or pressure exerted on the dorsal column. I use a series of tests to locate the site of the damage, using sensory stimulation to find out which level of the dorsal column has incurred an injury.

Bone is an excellent conductor of vibration and is therefore capable of resonance. The fact that each vertebra in the spine has a characteristic shape means that each vertebra has a separate and distinct resonant frequency. If the bones of the spine lose their position, the harmonic waves traveling up and down the spine are interrupted. This can lead to an exaggeration or lessening of the curves of the spine, which in turn affects the stability and flexibility of the spine and the integrity of the nervous system.

Vibratory sensation should be perceived equally on both sides of the body. Decreased vibratory sense on one side may indicate decreased brain function depending on the correlation of other findings.

Pinwheel Sensation: The pinwheel is used to test pain sensation and compare the feeling from side to side to make sure the nerve cells of the body are responding as they should. Sensory receptors account for our ability to see, hear, taste, and smell, and to sense touch, pain, temperature, and body position. The sensitivity of a sensory receptor usually depends on how much it has recently been stimulated. Hence, if a receptor like a nerve fiber in the skin is exposed to a constant stimulus, such as pressure on the skin, the rate of nerve impulses quickly falls to a much lower level, or even ceases altogether. This phenomenon is called adaptation and leads receptors to be more sensitive to changing than to steady stimulation.

This is why it's important to test almost every part of the skin with the pinwheel. The sensors on both sides of the body should react equally in sensitivity – if they don't, it may mean I need to dig a little deeper to find out why.

Muscle Strength: I find it amusing the scientists and those in charge of the medical language system seem to come up with long words for such simple things, like muscle strength testing. Kinesiology is the medical term used for muscle movement and is based on the idea that your body knows what's wrong with it, if you know how to listen.

The underlying principle is that the body is run by chemical and electrical signals that are sent from the brain to the spinal cord and the nervous system. All of our organs are controlled by the brain and nervous system, and our hundreds of muscles are controlled by; and connected to the nervous system. If there's an interference with electrical messages, the result is a weakened muscle. A healthy muscle is naturally strong and will resist average resistance. What you probably think of as simple muscle strength is actually a much deeper connection to nerves, organs, glands and all of the systems of the body.

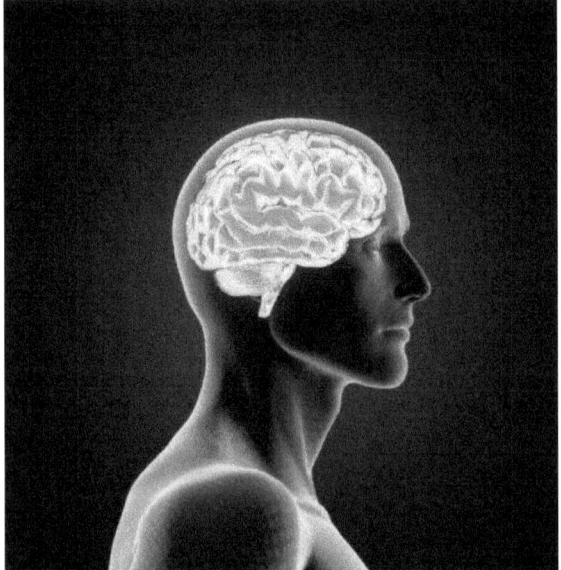

The nervous system is considered the master control and communication center of the body. It is responsible for regulating and maintaining body homeostasis or well-being. One of the functions of the nervous system is to cause a response called "motor output", which activates our muscles in response to sensory inputs received by the nervous system. An example of this would be like seeing a stop sign while driving and putting your foot on the brake pedal in response. Seeing the stop sign would be the sensory input and pressing the brake pedal would be the motor output. Because of the association between sensory input and muscle response, the development of muscle testing was born.

In a healthy body, each side of the body reacts equally in the same way. If they don't, it may mean I need to dig a little deeper to find out why. When the muscle response is weaker on one side of the body than the other, it may indicate that there is a short circuit in the neuromuscular signal, in other words, a weak nerve to muscle connection and no energetic balance related to the access point being tested.

Eye Exam: You've heard that the eyes are the window to the soul, but you may not have been told the eyes are also the window to the brain. It's amazing what can be seen by simply looking into the eyes of another person, if you know what to look for – and I do – and it's much more complex than what meets the eye.

We walk down a street, step up and down curbs, maneuver around objects and other pedestrians and adjust our pace, while visually monitoring our position. Moments later we get into our car, drive at highway speed through traffic and judge where we are relative to other vehicles while anticipating the flow of traffic. We arrive at baseball practice where we pick up a bat, walk to the plate, miss a curve ball, foul-off a fast ball and then hit a single, making numerous conscious and subconscious judgments with varying degrees of success.

After practice, we stop by the mall, scan the crowd for our friend, and go to the bookstore to find the book we might want to purchase. Over a no-foam latte, we read the opening chapter of this book, seeing if it captures our attention. This means the eyes and the brain are making the proper connections. By seeing this book, picking it up, opening the cover and reading your brain is working as it should thanks to your eyes. Sometimes, that's not the case.

An eye exam is done to check how someone's nervous system is functioning, especially after an injury or during illness. An eye exam would be abnormal if the pupils are:

- Pupils not of equal size

- Pupils not round or misshapen

- Pupils don't change when a light is shined on them as they should get smaller

- Pupils don't change when looking at something close or faraway.

The normal pupil constricts when either exposed directly to bright light or when that same light is presented to the other eye, referred to as the consensual response. This is due to the fact that stimulation of the nerves in one eye will activate and subsequently constriction of the pupils of both eyes. Disease or trauma of the brain will affect either the nerves associated with those limbs and will alter these responses accordingly. Also, strokes, brain tumors, collections of blood and more can result in dilatation of the pupils and unresponsiveness to direct stimulation by light.

As you can see, the eyes react in a very set, predictive way when stimulated. The way the eyes react, or fail to react, is therefore predictive of injury of some form to the brain or brain stem. When examining a patient's eyes, PERRLA is an acronym I use to describe the look and function of the eyes. It stands for:

➤ Pupils

➤ Equal

➤ Round

➤ Reactive to;

➤ Light and;

> ➢ Accommodation - This just means the ability of the
> eyes to focus on objects that are close-up and faraway.

Consensual Eye Movement: I will instruct a patient to watch
an object as it is brought towards the nose. The eyes then
actually converge towards the nose. If one eye moves out,
this may indicate decreased brain function on the same side.

Rapid Eye Movement between Two Specific Points: Rapid eye
movement between two specific points is assessed by having
the patient look from one finger held at mid-body to the finger
on the outside edge back and forth, as quickly as possible.
Saccadic eye movements, also referred to as saccades, are
rapid movements that move the eye from one object to the
next. Decreased speed or coordination in moving to one side
to the other may indicate decreased cerebellar function in the
opposite side or decreased brain function on the same side.
This could be indicative of disease, stroke, blood clots, nerve
damage and more.

Optokinetic tape: The Optokinetic Reflex can be tested by
passing an optokinetic tape in front of the patient's eyes, first
in one direction and then in the other, and observing the
motion of the eyes as the tape is passed. The saccadic
reflexes can also be tested by holding an optokinetic tape
about 14 inches from the eyes, and moving the tape slowly
and steadily first in one direction and then the other direction.
Any abnormality could be indicative of disease, stroke, blood
clots, nerve damage and more.

Olfactory Testing: Anything could smell as sweet as a rose –
as long as you can smell, right? You would be surprised
sometimes. Alzheimer's disease, Parkinson's disease, past

trauma to the brain and more can be diagnosed by olfactory testing.

The ability to smell, like everything else in the body, is a very simple yet highly complex set of processes in which several nerves play a major role. Sense of smell depends on the functioning of not only of cranial nerve 1 or the olfactory nerve, but also the positions of cranial nerve V called the trigeminal nerve.

Lack of smell on one side could also mean an under-performance on either the same side or opposite side of the cerebellum.

Diagnosis may easily lead to treatment of an underlying cause for the disturbance. Remember, many types of smell and taste disorders are reversible.

Facial Muscles and Associated Nerve Testing: Nerves not only control movement but rigidness and drooping of those muscles as well. The brain tells the facial nerve which muscles to move. The signal travels from the brain to the facial nerve. The nerve then splits into numerous branches along the face leading to the eyes, lips, cheeks, jaws, etc. The muscles control facial movements and expressions like eye blinking, smiling, frowning and more. Things like disease, past surgeries, accidents and trauma and more can affect your facial nerves and muscles.

The facial nerve resembles an electric cable and contains hundreds of individual nerve fibers. Each nerve fiber carries electrical impulses to a specific facial muscle. The facial nerve has several functions; however its main function is to move the muscles of the face, providing facial expression. In addition to carrying nerve impulses to the salivary and tear glands, it sends impulses to a muscle in the middle ear, which is attached to the stapes, the smallest bone in the middle ear. The facial nerve also has special fibers that provide taste to the tip of the tongue and pain fibers arising from the ear canal. As a result of facial nerve fibers being involved with different structures and different sites, disorders of the facial nerve may result in twitching, weakness or paralysis of the face, dryness of the eye or the mouth, loss of taste, increased sensitivity to loud sound, and pain in the ear.

Problems with the facial nerve may indicate decreased function in the opposite or the same side of the cerebellum.

What are the physical consequences of facial weakness caused by nerve inhibition, disease or trauma?

- Facial muscle weakness

- Facial sagging

- Inability to close the eyelid – can lead to eye injuries

- Difficulty chewing and drinking

- Drooling, because of weakness around the mouth

- Sensitivity to light, because the eyelids do not close

- Difficulty speaking, because the side of the face is sagging

- Appearance from asymmetry is very striking and can lead to depression

This is why it is so important to test these nerves and muscles. Bell's palsy, the beginning of Parkinson's disease and many other disorders can be identified through this simple yet important series of tests.

Testing the Cerebellum: The brain is comprised of a series of tissue layers - within those layers are formed structures which are made of different types of tissue: each structure serving a separate but distinct purpose. One of those structures is called the cerebellum. It lies under the cerebrum, towards the back, behind and above the brainstem.

The cerebellum is largely involved in coordination and oxygenation. Persons whose cerebellum doesn't work well are generally clumsy and unsteady. They may look like they are drunk even when they are not. Among many other things, activity in the cerebellum is essential for:

➢ The control of walking movements,

➢ The ability to maintain an upright posture,

➢ Fine-muscle coordination in skilled actions such as juggling objects or shuffling a deck of cards.

The largest part of the cerebellum is devoted to the coordination and control of habits. A habit is a coordinated sequence of automatic movements that has been learned through practice. When performing a habitual action such as shifting gears in a car with a manual transmission, we generally are not aware of the separate movements involved.

For some habits, it may be virtually impossible to become aware of the separate movements because they happen so quickly, and when we try to focus attention on them, the movements may become uncoordinated, thereby causing us to make mistakes.

If you focus attention on the separate movements involved in signing your name on a piece of paper, for example, you may notice that the resulting signature looks different from the way it looks when you're not paying attention. Habits typically are developed as the result of slow and deliberate practice, such as the long hours spent practicing a musical instrument or training for a sport like I did baseball. This practice causes changes in the cerebellum and in other areas of the brain — changes that underlie the development of the habit. Damage to the cerebellum often makes it difficult or impossible to learn new movements.

The role of the cerebellum in the production of habitual actions involves the adjustment of these movements to the specifics of a particular situation. For example, it is impossible to learn precisely how you should move in order to hit a baseball each time you step up to the plate: pitchers throw different pitches, the wind is blowing differently, you may be using a different bat, etc. Each time you step up to the plate, in order to swing the bat correctly, you must adjust your stance, your grip, your body posture, etc., to the changing circumstances.

This set of complex adjustments to a particular situation and the coordination of these adjustments — the "fine-tuning" of the habit — requires a great deal of activity in the cerebellum. Damage to the cerebellum can make it virtually impossible to adapt habitual movements in changing circumstances. This is why alcohol, which affects the cerebellum very quickly, can cause intoxicated people to appear so clumsy. In fact, people with damage to particular areas of the cerebellum may appear to be drunk for example, in Huntington's disease.

The cerebellum also may be involved in some higher mental functions: people with damage to the cerebellum sometimes show severe impairments in intellectual functioning. For example, they are more likely to have difficulty with planning actions and using language. Some of these impairments are due to difficulties in the ability to shift attention to new information. For example, most of us, while driving a car, would be able to easily shift our attention from a song on the radio to a weaving car ahead of us.

People with damage to the cerebellum, however, tend to have trouble doing this. The cerebellums of people with autism, for example, tend to show damage linked to attentional impairments in changing situations, especially social situations. In short, we can think of the cerebellum as being important not only for the coordination of movements in constantly changing situations but also for the coordination of attention in constantly changing situations.

Your brain and nervous system need two things to survive: fuel and activation. Fuel comes in the form of sugars called glucose and oxygen. You get the glucose from the food you eat but as you age, your ability to utilize oxygen decreases.

The cerebellum is the most dependent area of the body when it comes to oxygen. When the cerebellum is not firing correctly, the muscles will spasm, the vertebra lock up and the disc will lose fluid and degenerate. When I get the cerebellum firing better, everything simply functions and heals better because the essential body nutrients like sugars and oxygen are restored.

Some of the tests we do to access this part of the brain are:

Finger nose finger test: You stand with your eyes closed and are asked to touch your nose with your index finger - then open your eyes and touch my finger. If you cannot do this, it may indicate decreased cerebellar function on the same side.

Piano: Patients are asked to raise their arms straight out and pretend to play the piano as fast they possibly can with all of the fingers. What we are looking for differences from side-to-side. Any slow or more deliberate movement of one side versus the other would indicate decreased cerebellar function on that side.

Supination/pronation: Patients are asked to hold their hands straight out and asked to turn the hands upside down - and then right side up as fast as they can repeatedly. We are looking for any slow or deliberate movement one side versus the other which would indicate cerebellar dysfunction on that side.

Heel-to-toe walk: The patient walks in a straight line with heel touching the toe on every step, like you were taking a sobriety test. Unsteadiness or imbalance would indicate cerebellar dysfunction.

Romberg's test: This checks evaluation of the integrity of dorsal columns of the spinal cord. This simple test offers an important clue to the presence of disease in the nerve pathway. Early detection of reversible causes is the goal so we can prevent permanent dysfunction and disability.

Parietal Lobe Testing: The parietal lobes can be divided into two functional regions. One involves sensation and perception and the other is concerned with integrating sensory input, primarily with the visual system. The first function integrates sensory information to form a single perception called cognition. The second function constructs a spatial system to represent and help us make sense of the world around us. Individuals with damage to the parietal lobes often show striking deficits, such as abnormalities in body image and spatial relations.

Damage to the left parietal lobe can result in what is called "Gerstmann Syndrome." It includes right-left confusion, difficulty with writing and difficulty with mathematics. It can also produce disorders of language and the inability to perceive objects normally.

Damage to the right parietal lobe can result in neglecting part of the body or space, which can impair many self-care skills such as dressing and washing. Right side damage can also cause difficulty in drawing ability. Deficits primarily to memory and personality can occur if there is damage to the area between the parietal and temporal lobes.

A simple test in which you stand with your feet together, eyes closed and hands straight out can tell me many things. If one arm drifts and the other arm doesn't, that would possibly indicate parietal lobe dysfunction.

Temporal Lobe Testing: The temporal lobes are involved in the primary organization of sensory input and can be damaged by trauma, disease or stroke.

Language can be affected by temporal lobe damage. Left temporal trauma or disease affect and disturb the recognition of words. Right temporal damage can cause a loss of inhibition of talking. The temporal lobes are highly associated with memory skills.

Seizures of the temporal lobe can have dramatic effects on an individual's personality. Temporal lobe epilepsy can cause speech outbursts, paranoia and aggressive rages. Severe damage to the temporal lobes can also alter sexual behavior.

Common tests for temporal lobe function are: Rey-Complex Figure evaluating visual memory and Wechsler Memory Scale - Revised evaluates verbal memory. I will ask you to repeat back to me seven numbers. The inability to repeat those numbers or if spoken back in a monotone voice indicates decreased left temporal lobe function. The inability to repeat the numbers if broken or in a rhythmic variation, indicates decreased right temporal lobe function.

Neurologic Specific Treatments & Brain Based Therapy

How many brains do you have - one or two? While you have only one brain, the cerebral hemispheres are divided right down the middle into a right hemisphere and a left hemisphere. Each hemisphere is specialized for some behaviors. The right side of the brain controls muscles on the left side of the body and the left side of the brain controls muscles on the right side of the body. Also, in general, sensory information from the left side of the body crosses over to the right side of the brain and information from the right side of the body crosses over to the left side of the brain. Therefore, damage to one side of the brain will affect the opposite side of the body. Now, you can see why it's so important for both halves of the brain to work in harmony with each other.

Sometimes, either because of trauma suffered from playing football early in life, car accidents, falls, sickness or disease – these brain halves stop communicating like they should with one another. The aforementioned testing will indicate any decreased or uneven function on either side of the brain. Now you can see that the proper evaluation is very important to specifically identify any neurological problems. The reason I say this is because proper treatment is needed to restore things back to the way they once were.

Proper treatment is needed for what? Many if not all of these nightmarish conditions that you have, also have a neurological component to it which creates an imbalance in function of the right brain versus left brain hemispheres. If that is the case then the "neurological loop" of body to brain and back to the body needs to be addresses and remedied. Let me give you an example of the neurological loop.

Say for instance that you have a disc herniation as described earlier which is creating chronic and disabling pain. That nasty disc is sending signals from the nervous system up into the cerebellum portion of the brain. The cerebellar portion of the brain is firing to the opposite part of the brain. Now, the brain sends signals to the lower two-thirds of the brain stem. One of the functions of the lower two-thirds of the brain stem is to control the impulses directly to the remaining upper one-third of the brain stem known as the "mesencephalon". The mesencephalon many times, because of these chronic conditions, over-fires electrical signals through the nerves, right down through the spinal cord then back to those areas of pain and disease – and that is what is known as the neurological loop.

If this is not addressed neurologically, then that neurological loop is going to continue; over and over and over, hence your "chronic" condition and low back disability, dysfunction, and pain. The same is true with other chronic conditions such as fibromyalgia, carpal tunnel syndrome, insomnia/lack of sleep, migraine/chronic headache, peripheral neuropathy, restless legs syndrome, sciatica, multiple sclerosis compensation symptoms, vertigo or dizziness, tinnitus and balance problems.

Brain Based Therapy is a unique approach used to pinpoint and treat both past and current physical, chemical and emotional traumas which is responsible for aberrant neurological function. By utilizing brain stimulating modalities such as vibration, auricular stimulation to the ear; sound and smell stimulation, eye exercises and visual stimulation; I can activate specific sides of the brain that may be under-firing.

Stimulating specific sides utilizing gentle manipulation procedures to one side of the upper cervical spine functionally normalizes your nervous system. This area is a primary window into the nervous system. Additionally, I address brain fuel requirements in the form of diet and nutritional supplementation.

These treatment methods are some of the most powerful techniques known to reverse fibromyalgia and chronic pain.

However, only a small number of doctors in the U.S., 500 or so are utilizing them!

Severe and long-term stress on the body develops into a neurological pattern that often becomes damaging to the nervous system. This neurological pattern or stress response can become chronic and lead to chronic pain syndromes because fibers in the body that feel pain get inappropriately "turned on" and feel pain considerably more than the average person.

Fibromyalgia is a good example of this and the longer you have it the more and faster your brain dies. The electrical impulse continues to loop over and over and in like any form of circuitry, sooner than later it will wear out. This can also cause:

- Episodes of depression/anxiety

- Difficulty scanning pages while reading

- Difficulty adding or subtracting

- Difficulty expressing what you want to say

- Difficulty understanding what others say to you

- Loss of short or long term memory/ problems focusing

- Changes in handwriting

- More irritable or angry moods

- Problems with balance, tripping or dropping things

- Learning disabilities like dyslexia, ADD, ADHD

There are treatments and brain based therapies for the above conditions, and more. Let's take a look at some of the more common treatments and therapies I administer.

Unilateral Manipulation: General joint manipulation is used on one side of the body to stimulate nerve receptors on the cerebellar dysfunction side. Very gentle instrumentation may be used to accomplish this such as the ArthroStim® and VibraCussor®. The ArthroStim® Instrument works on the principle of neurological feedback. The partial dislocation pattern of joint stiffness, pain and muscle spasm results in altered sensory input from all the sensitive nerve receptors in joints, ligaments, muscles, tendon and skin. The ArthroStim® delivers a powerful sensory barrage to the brain. Because the ArthroStim® oscillations are so rapid, they do not fire pain receptors so the treatment is comfortable and pain free. The powerful sensory input "resets" the postural programs in the brain, restoring normal function and position of the spine or extremity joint.

VibraCussor® percussive therapy is an exciting new treatment approach for muscle and ligament problems. The VibraCussor® delivers waves of percussive impulses deep into the tissues of the body which reach the muscles. VibraCussor® therapy is very effective for releasing muscles which have been tight and thus sore for prolonged periods. The VibraCussor® compression waves promote an increase in circulation and lymphatic fluid flow and a decrease in muscle spasm. This is great for those who participate in sports because the repetitive pumping action of the VibraCussor® is ideal for releasing adhesions. The power of multiple percussive waves accumulates to loosen up 'stuck' areas without using heavy thrusting forces. Additionally, these waves heighten neurological awareness of specific areas of the body.

These instruments are very beneficial to people suffering from migraine headaches, fibromyalgia, dizziness and chronic fatigue syndrome.

Dorsal Spine Manipulation: Thoracic adjustments – manipulation to the long middle part of the spine, are used to activate the dorsal column pathways. The dorsal column pathways need to be balanced to send proper electrical signals up to the cerebellar portion of the brain which we talked about earlier. This also increases the "tidal volume", or the overall amount of air in the lungs. As you will remember, the cerebellar portion of the brain is the most oxygen dependent structure of the body so to improve brain balance, improve brain function, increased oxygenation is very important.

Dorsal spine manipulation is recommended, or is an option, for a number of disorders, including acute and chronic low back pain, neck pain and some types of headache.

In practice, manipulation is also used in the management of extremity joint disorders for complaints such as carpal tunnel syndrome, and shoulder, ankle, knee, and hip pain.

Upper and Lower Extremity Adjustment: The goal of the spinal adjustment is to restore normal movement and function to the joint and surrounding muscles. The nerves nearby can also be positively affected, helping with pain down the leg or even helping improve focus and cognitive function. When the joint is adjusted or realigned into its proper position, the joint and muscle move and function well, much like the ride of a car is smoother when the alignment is straight and the tires are rotated and balanced. The improved function of the joint causes a decrease in pain. Pain is usually not the main problem in the body, but rather a signal to the body that something is wrong. If the pain is caused by the joint misalignment or a compressed nerve, relieving the joint or nerve should relieve the pain.

When the joints are adjusted it will hurt less to sit up straight and the bones will also be in their proper positions. After an adjustment the joints in the spine or extremities can move more freely and in a larger or more normal range of motion. People who have pain do not move in a full range of motion, so decreasing the pain will also help to increase the range of motion.

When you are activating same side of the cerebellum, it is very important because it uses the feed-forward mechanism (remember the loop I spoke of) to the opposite side of the brain - and again depending on what we need to do to stimulate the nerve depends on the location at which we do these adjustments.

Auditory Stimulation: Sound therapy has existed in one form or another for many years. The current literature suggests that the right cerebral hemisphere is more sensitive to low frequency sounds and that the left cerebral hemisphere is more sensitive to high frequency sounds.

The left cerebral hemisphere is the dominant hemisphere for language in ninety-nine percent of right hand dominant people and ninety-six percent of left hand dominant people. The left cerebral hemisphere is commonly associated with being more sequential, analytical, detail oriented, and logical than the right hemisphere. The right hemisphere is more commonly associated with global processing, seeing images, perceiving shape and motion, and speech intonation. The "Mozart Effect" targets the left cerebral hemisphere as compositions by Mozart have some of the greatest occurrences of high frequency notes in them. Auditory stimulation in one ear increases the nerve impulses in the opposite side of the cerebral cortex.

Sound therapy has recently been shown to have a significant effect on postural stability. Different music can affect the activation of different parts of the brain (dorsolateral prefrontal cortex, occipital cortex, and cerebellum) differently. Maybe Mozart was right after all!

Visual Stimulation: Visual stimulation is a powerful therapy used to create neurological changes. Visual stimulation may take the form of shining a flashlight into one or both eyes, having the eyes move in specific directions, or giving the eyes specific visual targets to look at or watch. These stimulations are so varied because each section of the brain plays a different role in the processing of visual information.

The occipital lobe at the back of the brain is the primary visual area. The parietal lobe at the top of the brain tends to see things that move quickly, have low contrast, and which are below us. The parietal lobe also helps us to locate where an object is positioned and allows us to smoothly follow a moving target. The temporal lobe at the bottom of the brain tends to see things that move slowly, have high contrast, and are above us. The temporal lobe also helps us identify the object at which we are looking.

The frontal lobe is responsible for the fast eye movements we use when we acquire and look at a new target. The frontal lobe can generate eye movements up to 900 degrees per second, so all of these functions are integrated by the brainstem. Pictures of faces increases brain function via a feed-forward mechanism in the cerebellum to the cortex. By contrast, familiar faces will stimulate the left prefrontal cortex and unfamiliar faces will stimulate the right. It's interesting that observing only large letters will stimulate right hemisphere and right brain. Observing only small letters will stimulate the left hemisphere of the brain.

I give your brain a workout – literally. By applying this type therapy in conjunction with an overall treatment plan, your brain not only gets stronger, but your nerves relearn to function normally again.

TENS Physiotherapy: Everything in the medical field it seems has acronyms, abbreviations or three different names. This is why it takes so long to get through medical school! On a more serious note, you've heard of a TENS unit before I'm sure. TENS is an acronym for **T**ranscutaneous **E**lectrical **N**erve **S**timulator – it's a small package that delivers big results. This electrical stimulation is used at a very low setting to affect the same side cerebellum and opposite hemisphere of the brain.

Millions of people suffer from chronic pain conditions such as back pain, arthritis, joint pain, shingles and fibromyalgia. Various prescription drugs and treatments are used to fight chronic pain and I won't discount that, but sometimes pain killers are too strong for people leading an active life. The warnings on pain killers for "do not drive" and "do not use heavy equipment" prevent many people from driving and working – they are there for a good reason.

An alternative method used by professional athletes and people on the go, is a transcutaneous electrical nerve stimulator, or TENS physiotherapy. It works by sending electrical impulses to select parts of the body to block pain and increase the level of endorphins – those natural pain killers produced by the brain. The position of the electrodes on the skin determines which nerves are stimulated. Once the nerves are stimulated, the natural pain killers of the body can do what they are supposed to do.

Heat Therapy: Warmth and heat are usually associated with comfort and relaxation. But heat therapy goes a step further and can provide relief from the muscle spasm pain cycle and aid your body in healing itself. Heat Therapy is typically used for chronic pain that has no swelling. Chronic refers to an injury, illness or disease that develops slowly and is persistent and long lasting. Because the symptoms are often mild, they are often ignored or overlooked for months or years. It begins as a small nagging ache or pain and can grow into a debilitating injury if not treated early. Chronic injuries are also referred to as cumulative trauma, overuse injury, or repetitive stress injury.

Heat applications warm the tissue beneath it causing the veins to dilate and increasing blood flow. This results in an increase in metabolism, oxygen and nutrient supply. This reduces pain by slowing the nerves ability to send signals to the brain. Warming muscle fibers reduces their sensitivity and rate of firing, resulting in less spasm. Heat therapy also increases the extensibility of collagen tissue, making joints and muscles more flexible.

Intersegmental Traction: It sounds scary, but it's not. It's really very soothing. Although not actually a traction device, this table helps with blood flow and to reinforce the adjustments by creating additional movement to spinal joints. It's a table that rolls or massages the spine from underneath while you lie comfortably on your back and enjoy the experience! Remember the dorsal column; the back portion of the spinal cord which sends important information up to the cerebellum portion of the brain? This is what we stimulate here.

Intersegmental traction tables gently help reestablish the normal ranges of the body's spine. Intersegmental traction tables also help facilitate muscle relaxation and reduce muscle spasms. It has been shown that use of an intersegmental traction table greatly accelerates recovery progress from a back injury. The intersegmental table operates by a dual roller moving up and down the muscles on either side of the spine. The rolling contact is constant and works electronically. Intersegmental traction tables are very relaxing and make for a great healing tool.

Benefits:

*An intersegmental traction table mobilizes the spinal column while simultaneously and gently stretching ligaments and muscles.

*Intersegmental traction tables increase blood flow and the oxygen to discs in the back, ligaments and the muscles, thereby improving balance, strength and mobility.

Warm and Cold Caloric's: This treatment is very, very effective for my patients with vertigo, balance disorder, dizziness, migraine and chronic headaches. The semicircular canal is the portion of the inner ear and is responsible for position and balance sense. Inside that little semicircular canal, there are fluid and small hairs known as "stereocilia" and "kinocilia". The stereocilia and kinocilia literally send nerve impulse back to the cerebellum and therefore increases the firing to the same side cerebellum.

In time the fluid of the inner ear can turn into a sludge or soft gel like substance and because of that, does not move around within those canals like it once did. A warm caloric is inserting warm water into the external ear canal. This does not go into the brain. This bounces off of the eardrum and comes right back out, but the heated water liquefies the sludge or gel like fluid so that it can become completely fluid once again. When the ear fluid moves freely the chronic condition is improved. Cold caloric's use the exact opposite effect of the warm caloric. We use this when we want to decrease the frequency of the nerve impulses on the same side cerebellum and thus restore normalcy.

UBE: UBE stands for **U**pper **B**ody **E**rgometer: It's a bicycle for your arms. Instead of placing your feet on the bicycle pedals, you place your hand on specially positioned pedals and you move these pedals in a circular motion. This increases the nerve firing of the posterior or back group of muscles which includes the neck and arms. This in turn increases stimulation to the to the cerebellum also increasing its activation.

Remember earlier I pointed out there are two things needed for the brain to function at its utmost: One is fuel and the other is activation. Fuel for the body and brain comes in the forms of glucose and oxygen. Glucose is a sugar which comes from a proper diet. The second is oxygen. Increasing oxygen to the brain is very, very important to those patients suffering with chronic conditions, especially when pain is involved.

I already mentioned that the dorsal spinal adjustment is very important to increasing lung capacity. When you have increased lung capacity you have ability to increase the amount of oxygen dispersed to the body and then back to the brain. Upper body ergometers are important because they bring more blood flow and in turn oxygen towards the upper body and closer to the brain.

Meditation: Meditation is recommended to improve breath therefore increasing oxygenation to the brain. Earlier in this book I had mentioned some of the neurological testing such as oxygen saturation. Meditation actually helps with this.

Meditation is the practice of connecting with your inner self in an effort to release your mind from specific stress factors, anxieties or fears. Meditation is the ability to release negative energy within your body and mind, physically, mentally and oftentimes spiritually as well. The goal of meditation is to transform those negative energies into positive energy which can be used to act as healing benefits for the stress, anxiety, and fears. Meditation offers clarity and peace of mind. The medical benefits of meditation can result in healing for the three main areas of health: physical, mental and spiritual.

Olfactory Stimulation: Olfactory stimulation is used to increase the nerve impulses to the same side brain. This Improves frontal lobe activation which helps with various neurological disorders.

Remember, as discussed earlier, your brain controls and coordinates all function of the body. When functioning normally, the cerebellum sends messages or "fires" to the brain's right and left hemisphere, which in turn "fires" to the brain stem. This is called the "Brain Loop" I spoke of earlier in the book. Olfactory stimulation is stimulating your senses by smell – therefore stimulating your brain.

What steps can I take to help myself live a healthy, productive neurological lifestyle you ask?

That's a very good question and an easy one to answer. Let's look back at what we've discussed here and relate that to what you have access to at home.

Exercise: Muscles and joints need movement to function as they should. If you don't move it, you lose it. If you don't exercise, you actually lose oxygen to the brain.

Enjoy Life: Enjoy your senses! Music has various health benefits because of the way it enhances emotional responses in people. For a fitness routine, music can keep the body going and guide the rhythm of the workout. The benefit of listening to music while exercising is not reserved for those who are recovering from an illness. It can work for everyone because of the effect that music has on the brain's frontal lobe. To fully interpret the tones, sequences, and timing of music, the frontal lobe should be more active.

Don't forget your sense of smell! The smell of a lone Lilac tree can bring back a flood of memories. Just a single whiff can trigger parts of your brain to fire that may not have activated in decades. Plus when you get a whiff of something that causes your brain to fire, it stimulates your eyes. Say you smell lilacs, the very first thing you'll do is look around to see if you can identify the tree!

Speaking of the eyes – it's important to keep the eyes going as well. Big letters; small letters – various colors – combine those with music and a walk in the park or even your back yard and there you have it! While you're walking you can look around at all the faces you encounter. It's your very own neurological plethora of self-healing!

Testimonial

Patient: Betty Stefens

Chief Complaint Treated: Vertigo

I'll start by saying I fell in the kitchen. As a result, I ended up with a concussion. It even affected my smell (Who knew!). In about a week or so I noticed something was wrong. I was crying all the time and when I went to bed, I would wake with dizziness. The room would just spin and spin and the ceiling would flip over and over. My memory and my speech were also affected.

Dr. Coniglio treated me with Brain Based Therapy, something new. He explained Brain Based Therapy to me. I went for a cat scan to make sure I didn't have a brain bleed. (Result: no bleeding!) Within 4 weeks I was back to my old self again with the help of Dr. Coniglio and his staff! Thank you so much!

Chapter Five

Physical Testing and Treatment

S o many times patients have chronic, nightmarish conditions and are medicated for a period of years. Many of these patients have been through twenty or more medications over the decades and are still suffering with a worsening chronic condition. Many times there are multiple causes which lie within the metabolic, neurological and physical deficiencies a person develops over time. A detailed physical examination is needed in order to address the exact cause of the problem. We isolate the main cause of the chronic condition and if we can, we fix it.

Joints are where bones come together. Joints hold the bones together and allow for movement of the skeleton. All of the bones form joints. Joints are complex structures made up of many parts. The first thing we assess is range of motion. Flexion is how far the joint can be bent forward. Extension is how far it can be bent backward. Generally speaking, range of motion refers to the distance and direction a joint can move to its full potential. People with chronic conditions typically have lost significant range of motion.

It's important to know the normal range of motion for each joint. After physical examination, if it is determined that you

114

have limited or abnormal range of motion in one or more joints, we'll put together a treatment plan.

Reflexes: There are three very important spinal nerve reflexes in the neck which go into the arms to allow the nervous system to coordinate movement and there are two very important reflexes in the low back which coordinate function of the legs.

As I noted earlier, we also have to do the muscle stretch reflex responses. The muscle stretch reflex responses are the reflexes you exhibit when you are sitting and the doctor tests the patient's reflex with a medical hammer. We test for movement – and reflex response. If you have adequate movement and response that means that that nerve root is working sufficiently.

Orthopedic testing is to evaluate for structural integrity within the body. We perform 30 different orthopedic tests which give us the exact deficiency of the structures involved.

Muscle strength testing is important. We test the muscles manually. Manual muscle testing evaluates which muscles are strong versus weak, right versus left. We coordinate the muscular findings with the range of motion findings, neurologic findings and the chiropractic orthopedic findings.

Manipulative techniques: There are different manipulation techniques that are used to help increase range of motion. These manipulation techniques are performed in the spine as well as the extremities. Many methods complement each other and work best when combined. Each individual is different and therefore may respond better to one treatment more than another. Additionally, some people have a preference to the technique that is used in their treatment.

The first technique is called diversified technique. Diversified technique is a manual treatment of manipulation of the spine to increase range of motion at the spinal level for spinal loss. Diversified technique is an incorporation of many singular methods. Diversified technique stresses the integration of a detailed history and thorough biomechanical exam which involves both your nervous and musculoskeletal systems.

The treatment protocol may include adjustments, physiotherapeutic modalities, stretches, nutritional supplements, orthotics and other aids.

Thomson technique is a technique used with a specific table that has moveable devices that makes it easier for the patient to be adjusted. We use these tables if someone has severe muscle spasm where their muscles are so tight that it is very difficult to manipulate the spine - unless we have specific aids in doing so. The use of different tables offers us the ability to use different manipulative techniques to help attain the specific goals that are needed.

We utilize what is called "flexion distraction technique" with our flexion distraction table. The flexion distraction table is an adjusting table where the lower end of the table passively and mechanically moves up and down.

We allow the patient to lie in a specific position on this table and I place my hands on specific points of the body while the table is passively flexing and extending. This accomplishes many things. One, it increases movement of the area of the body. Second, it creates a pumping action. This pumping action is important because it helps literally pump that inflammation and swelling away from the injured area. We know that when swelling and inflammation is reduced an area will heal faster. Third, it increases the size of the foramen; the holes where the spinal nerves exit the spinal cord.

When closure of the foramen occurs in combination with chronic conditions, the patient typically has disc herniation, disc bulging and overly degenerative joint disease. These holes have been closed due to the aforementioned chronic conditions.

ArthroStim® Instrumentation: The ArthroStim® is an extension of our hands. The ArthroStim® introduces gentle force onto your body at 12-14 "taps" or cycles per second.

VibraCussor®: The VibraCussor® is a variable speed massage device which has different attachments to stimulate different body parts. The two major goals of the VibraCussor® are to increase oxygen going to the area that needs healing, and reduce chronic muscle spasm.

Electro-auricular Instrumentation: There are different acupuncture points on the ear that relate to different areas of the body which offer immense pain relief. We perform this electroacupuncture on most chronic condition patients with great success.

This amazing device applies the same principle as the age old Chinese therapy of acupuncture, without piercing the skin and then stimulates away the pain electronically at the touch of a button, without needles.

High-volt Muscular Stimulation: This electrical muscular stimulation device is a physiotherapy mechanism that provides an electrical current to the muscles. This reduces the amount of muscle spasm. This also helps reduce inflammation. This treatment is typically 15 minutes duration and is painless.

Intersegmental Traction: Intersegmental traction is a mechanical table which increases the range of motion of the spinal joints and is exactly as described earlier. The duration of this is 15 minutes.

Interferential Therapy: Interferential therapy is an electrical muscular stimulator to reduce muscle spasm as well as reduce inflammation at the injured site. It uses a mid-frequency current for treating muscular spasm and strains. The current produces a massaging effect over the affected area at periodic intervals, and this stimulates the secretion of endorphins; the body's natural pain relievers, thus relaxing the strained muscles and promoting soft-tissue healing. Treatment duration is 15 minutes.

Therapeutic Rehabilitation: Therapeutic rehabilitation is used in our office to specifically create a better balance with the flexibility and strength of an individual. First the patient is individually instructed on exercises to increase their flexibility. Once improved flexibility is attained, we gently graduate them to strengthening exercises. As strengthening improves we increase the demand of the exercises and overall strength improves.

Nonsurgical Spinal Decompression: Nonsurgical spinal decompression is a state of the art treatment for chronic conditions. This specialized treatment table was originally used for the chronic disc herniations, disc bulges, spinal stenosis, sciatic, and degenerative joint and disc disease. This very important, specialized piece of equipment is also helpful with other chronic conditions such as fibromyalgia, chronic fatigue syndrome, migraine headaches, and peripheral neuropathy.

Home Exercise Program (HEP): Home participation is very important in the successful treatment and ongoing successful elimination of pain. Independence is an important part of anyone's life. At some point, I will transition you into a home exercise program. Depending on the severity of the injury and extent of damage to your tissues, this may start very soon or occur later in the treatment program.

Exercises that will increase your flexibility, strength and balance are a natural progression to giving you an independent life. Strength and flexibility gains made during treatment in our office may be quickly lost if activity is not maintained. Our patients are instructed to perform a home exercise program as well as given specific instruction for modification of activities of daily living which make their lives better.

Testimonial

Patient: Donald Quinn

Chief Complaint Treated: Migraine Headache and Disc Bulges (No Surgery Needed due to Treatment)

Before starting with Dr. Coniglio, I was getting severe violent headaches almost twice a week as a result of bulging discs in my neck. These headaches were so painful they would sometimes immobilize me. I am unable to take medications they prescribed for pain.

Because these headaches were so severe, the day after I had one would be a wasted day because I had to recover from the pain of the previous day. I was also experiencing pain due to bulging discs in my back. I had been to the Rothman Institute and the University of Pennsylvania and both suggested surgery.

After a period of time of seeing Dr. Coniglio, my back started to feel better and my neck issues started to improve. As of today, my headaches are not nearly as frequent or severe. I am able to do things I previously could not and my quality of life is much improved. The most important thing is that the headaches and back pain have subsided substantially.

I would share (with friends and family members) that I had been to two previous chiropractors and was skeptical about going to another one. I was against any kind of surgery. After a few visits with Dr. Coniglio, I started to feel better. I would suggest that they give it a try and stick with it. The staff is very helpful and informative (and) Dr. Coniglio answers questions in a very down to earth manner and explains the condition of my neck and back, and what is needed to improve it.

120

Chapter Six

The Keys to Healing

We help the absolute worst of the worst patients get better because we are comprehensive and flexible. That is the reason our treatments are successful at stopping these chronic nightmarish conditions in their tracks. This really means a lot to me, to be able to serve you the gracious reader, through a book like this and I'd like to take a moment and tell you about what the words I have chosen means to me personally.

The word "comprehensive" is very important because we combine the metabolic, neurologic, and physical treatment inside that category. Most doctors are specialists and only test and treat for metabolic - or only test and treat for neurologic - or only test and treat for physical. Our comprehensive evaluation and treatment includes all three because we treat the whole person – not just part of you or your body.

Let me talk about the word "flexibility". When I talk about flexibility, I do not only mean flexibility in your muscles. What I mean by that, simply put, our treatment can change from visit to visit depending upon your needs. We are not locked into treatment protocol for four week periods like most specialties. Having flexibility to serve your needs at any time and change treatment modalities if needed provides a better outcome. That is the beauty of this treatment. It is tailor made just for you as an individual, and is very flexible to try to get you better in the shortest period of time possible.

When combining these treatments, most patients see some, if not complete resolution of their condition.

We are all creatures of habit and change is one of the most difficult things in life to implement, especially if you feel like you are the only one that must change. We are fooling ourselves if we don't take the time needed to heal. I don't mean sitting on the couch all day and watching the world pass by while you eat potato chips, I mean changing a lifestyle that brought your body into the aches, pains and disease which now forces you to modify your life, and from that come into a lifestyle which brings health, healing, happiness and acceptance. It's all in how you look at things-----being positive or being negative and continually thinking about all the things that you "can't" do when there are so many more things you "can" do!

I have noticed that there is a different agenda going on with regard to what we think we want as far as healing our bodies is concerned, and what our inner-self seems to want. Its agenda seems to be for us to achieve the greater plan for our life - which does include negative things that will force us, hopefully to reconnect with our inner selves and our sense of physical well-being.

One of the reasons our practice has been so successful, is because I am firmly committed to helping you wash away the negative – the pain and suffering – and I want so bad to see you start living and enjoying life again. If you'll let me, I'll help you.

Thank you so much for allowing me to come into your home and life.

Chapter Seven

Self-Help Low Impact Stretches & Exercises

As I mentioned, exercises can help lessen that nagging backache. They strengthen and stretch muscles that support the back and legs and promote good posture— keeping the muscles of the back, abdomen, hips, and upper body strong. They can also keep you mobile and limber – and that's important.

Exercises will also help ease back pain and help prepare you for labor and delivery. Staying active during pregnancy can help with back pain.

Here I'm including some mild stretches and exercises and almost anyone can do that will help keep you active and limber.

Seniors

Exercises and stretches can improve your strength and mobility -- and help you get back to your usual routine. You can do some exercises if you're still using a wheelchair or walker.

Arm Strengthener

This exercise builds your arm muscles even if you don't have the strength to lift yourself out of a chair, according to the National Institutes of Health. Sit in a chair that has arms and lean forward a little, with your back straight. Grab the arms of the chair. Lift your heels up so your weight is on the balls of your feet. Using your hands -- not your legs -- push yourself as high off the chair as you can. Return to sitting, rest a few seconds and do a total of 10 repetitions.

> **Disclaimer: Before you start any exercise or stretching program, consult with your health care provider. Your health care provider can give you personal exercise guidelines, based on your medical history.**

Hand Squeeze

After a hospital stay, strengthen your grip with the hand squeeze exercise, recommended by the University of Georgia. Sit up straight in a chair and hold a rubber ball in front of your stomach. Have one hand on each side of the ball, with your fingers spread out. Press the ball as if you were trying to squeeze the air out of it. Hold for four seconds and release your hands slowly. Do a total of eight repetitions, rest and do another eight.

Waist Bends

Ohio State University Medical Center recommends this exercise for rehabilitation after a heart attack. Stand with your feet shoulder-distance apart. Place your hands on your hips. With your legs and back straight, bend to your right as far as you comfortably can. Return to your starting position and repeat to your left. Do a total of 10 repetitions.

Arm Raises

This arm exercise also provides cardiovascular rehabilitation, according to Ohio State University. Stand with your feet shoulder-distance apart and your arms hanging at your sides. With elbows straight, slowly lift your arms in front of you and up in the air as far as you comfortably can. Slowly drop your arms, pause and repeat. Do a total of 10 repetitions.

Isometric Exercises

Isometric exercises are relatively low impact exercises that help maintain strength in muscle groups. There are many isometric exercises you can do at home with very little equipment that will produce great results.

Isometric exercises are not necessarily the type of exercise you want to perform for increasing your muscle mass. Nor will isometric exercises increase strength. These exercises are great for relieving injury-related pain, such as tendonitis, and for stretching.

Flexion

Stand with a wall or doorway on one side of your body. Make a fist and place your forearm against the wall so it is flush with the wall up to the inside of your elbow. Push against the wall for a few seconds. Switch sides and repeat with the other arm.

External Rotation

Stand perpendicular to a wall and bend your elbow to a 90 degree angle. Make a fist with your hand and place the side of your forearm against the wall. Press toward the wall and hold this position for a few seconds before switching sides to perform the exercise with the other arm.

Hands on Head

Not all isometric exercises need props. You can perform rehabilitation or stretching for your neck just by using your hands. Clasp your hands behind your head with your elbows bent and parallel to your shoulders. Press your head against your hands and press your hands against your head. Hold for a few seconds and release.

One Hand on Head

Perform side to side isometric exercises with one hand on the side of your head. Place your right palm on the right side of your head just above your ear. Press against your head with your hand as you press against your hand with your head. Hold for a few seconds, then switch sides.

As you can see, these exercises don't offer the weight and resistance necessary to build muscle or act as a stimulating cardiovascular routine. However, if you want to augment your stretching and warm up routine prior to your workout each day, isometric exercises will help keep you limber and assist you in maintaining healthy muscles.

Stretching Exercises for Pregnancy

Stretching exercise make the muscles limber and warm which can be especially helpful when you're pregnant. Here are some simple stretches you can perform before or after exercise.

Neck rotation

Relax your neck and shoulders. Drop your head forward. Slowly rotate your head to your right shoulder, back to the middle, and over the left shoulder. Complete four, slow rotations in each direction.

Shoulder rotation

Bring your shoulders forward and then rotate them up toward your ears and then back down. Do four rotations in each direction.

Swim

Place your arms at your sides. Bring your right arm up and extend your body forward and twist to the side, as if swimming the crawl stroke. Follow with left arm. Do the sequence ten times.

Thigh shift

Stand with one foot about two feet in front of the other, toes pointed in the same direction. Lean forward, supporting your weight on the forward thigh. Change sides and repeat. Do four on each side.

Leg Shake

Sit with your legs and feet extended. Move the legs up and down in a gentle shaking motion.

Ankle rotation

Sit with your legs extended and keep your toes relaxed. Rotate your feet, making large circles. Use your whole foot and ankle. Rotate four times on the right and four times on the left.

Kegel Exercises during Pregnancy

Kegel exercises help strengthen the muscles that support the bladder, uterus, and bowels. By strengthening these muscles during your pregnancy, you can develop the ability to relax and control the muscles in preparation for labor and birth. Kegel exercises are also highly recommended during the postpartum period to promote the healing of perineal tissues, increase the strength of the pelvic floor muscles and help these muscles return to a healthy state, and also increase urinary control.

To do Kegels, imagine you are trying to stop the flow of urine or trying not to pass gas. When you do this, you are contracting the muscles of the pelvic floor and are practicing Kegel exercises. While doing Kegel exercises, try not to move your leg, buttock, or abdominal muscles. In fact, no one should be able to tell that you are doing Kegel exercises. So you can do them anywhere!

I recommend doing five sets of Kegel exercises a day. Each time you contract the muscles of the pelvic floor, hold for a slow count of five and then relax. Repeat this ten times for one set of Kegels.

Tailor Exercises for Pregnancy

Tailor exercises strengthen the pelvic, hip, and thigh muscles and can help relieve low back pain.

Tailor sit

Sit on the floor with your knees bent and ankles crossed. Lean slightly forward, and keep your back straight but relaxed. Use this position whenever possible throughout the day.

Tailor press

Sit on the floor with your knees bent and the bottoms of your feet together. Grasp your ankles and pull your feet gently toward your body. Place your hands under your knees. Inhale. While pressing your knees down against your hands, press your hands up against your knees (counter-pressure). Hold for a count of five.

Stretches you can do at Work

Wrist Stretch

Extend arm in front, palm up and grab the fingers with other hand. Gently pull the fingers towards you to stretch the forearm, holding for 20-30 seconds. Repeat on the other side.

Wrist & Forearm

Press hands together in front of chest, elbows bent and parallel to the floor. Gently bend wrists to the right and left for 10 reps.

Lower Back Stretch

Sit tall and place the left arm behind left hip. Gently twist to the left, using the right hand to deepen the stretch, holding for 20-30 seconds. Repeat on the other side.

Hip Flexion

Sit tall with the abs in and lift the left foot off the floor a few inches, knee bent. Hold for 2 seconds, lower and repeat for 16 reps. Repeat on the other side.

Leg Extension

Sit tall with the abs in and extend the left leg until it's level with hip, squeezing the quadriceps. Hold for 2 seconds, lower and repeat for 16 reps. Repeat on the other side.

Inner Thigh

Place towel, firm water bottle or an empty coffee cup between the knees as you sit up tall with the abs in. Squeeze the bottle or cup, release halfway and squeeze again, completing 16 reps of slow pulses.

Chair Exercises

Chair Squat

While sitting, lift up until your hips are just hovering over the chair, arms out for balance. Hold for 2-3 seconds, stand all the way up and repeat for 16 reps.

Dips

Make sure chair is stable and place hands next to hips. Move hips in front of chair and bend the elbows, lowering the body until the elbows are at 90 degrees. Push back up and repeat for 16 reps.

One-Leg Squat

Make sure the chair is stable and take one foot slightly in front of the other. Use the hands for leverage as you push up into a one-legged squat, hovering just over the chair and keeping the other leg on the floor for balance. Lower and repeat, only coming a few inches off the chair for 12 reps. Repeat on the other side.

Upper Body Exercises

Front Raise to Triceps Press

Sit tall with the abs in and hold a full water bottle in the left hand. Lift the bottle up to shoulder level, pause, and then continue lifting all the way up over the head. When the arm is next to the ear, bend the elbow, taking the water bottle behind you and contracting the triceps. Straighten the arm and lower down, repeating for 12 reps on each arm.

Bicep Curl

Hold water bottle in right hand and, with abs in and spine straight, curl bottle towards shoulder for 16 reps. Repeat other side.

Abdominal Exercises

Side Bends

Hold a water bottle with both hands and stretch it up over the head, arms straight. Gently bend towards the left as far as you can, contracting the abs. Come back to center and repeat to the right. Complete 10 reps (bending to the right and left is one rep).

Ab Twists

Hold the water bottle at chest level and, keeping the knees and hips forward, gently twist to the left as far as you comfortably can, feeling the abs contract. Twist back to center and move to the left for a total of 10 reps. Don't force it or you may end up with a back injury.

Back strengthening Exercises

As shown in this book, your back is a complicated mechanical system with many moving parts. This is why the condition of the surrounding muscles is so important in supporting it and holding everything in alignment. Studies have shown the muscles that provide support to your back behave differently to other muscles. The key difference is that they are slower to automatically "switch back on" (i.e. return to their previous level of function) after an injury or a strain. Unless they are triggered by exercise, they can take a long time to return to their previous level of function.

Worst case without the right exercise, they may never return to full function and so your back doesn't get the support it needs. When these supporting muscles are working properly, they respond to signals from your brain by clenching or bracing fractionally before a strain impacts your back. This means your back is supported as the strain arrives and so the chance of (further) injury or strain is reduced.

When this mechanism is not working properly and the muscles don't trigger, your back is left unsupported and thus you are more likely to re-injure or strain your back. This is why back problems can be so difficult to get rid of once you start having them and why you can suffer from recurring back problems. This is also the reason regular exercise is so important - it helps to keep your supporting muscles active and able to do their job.

Here are nine back-strengthening exercises you can do at home -- stretching and flexion exercises to increase flexibility, and extension exercises to strengthen the muscles needed to counteract the force of gravity.

Stretching and Flexion Exercises -- To strengthen an acutely injured back, start with stretching and flexion exercises. These exercises increase flexibility and strength in the hip and lower back and in the abdominal and buttock muscles.

Abdominal Curl

Lie on your back with knees bent, feet flat on the floor, and your hands clasped lightly behind your head. Without pulling with your hands, slowly curl your shoulder blades up off the floor, leaving your back on the floor. Hold for five seconds and slowly lower your head and shoulders. Start with five repetitions, increasing the number by five as the curls get easier.

Knee Pull (Without/With Head Curl)

Lie on your back with knees bent and feet flat on the floor. Bring one knee up toward your chest and clasp the knee with both hands. Hold for 10–15 seconds. Return the leg to the starting position and repeat with the other leg. Start with three repetitions and then increase gradually by one every other day until you reach 12 repetitions. Once you can do that easily, add in a head curl. While you are holding your knee for 10–15 seconds, gently curl your head up slightly, then return to the starting position. Gradually work your way up to 12 repetitions.

Hurdler Stretch

While standing, place a chair or bench about three feet in front of you. Put the heel of one foot on the seat of the chair or the bench. Now bend forward at the waist and move your forehead toward your knee. Hold for 10–15 seconds. Return to the starting position and repeat with the other leg. Start with three repetitions and then increase gradually by one every other day until you reach 12 repetitions.

Pelvic Tilt

Lie on your back with knees bent and feet flat on the floor. Relax your back muscles, tighten your abdominal and buttock muscles, and press your back flat against the floor. This will tilt your pelvis forward. Once you have a totally flat back, hold the position for 10–15 seconds. Start with three repetitions and then increase gradually by one every other day until you reach 12 repetitions.

Modified Toe-touch

While standing with your feet hip-width apart, bend forward, bringing the top of your head toward the floor, and look backward between your knees. Go as far as you can and then grasp behind your knees and try to go a little farther. Hold for 10–15 seconds. Start with three repetitions and then increase gradually by one every other day until you reach 12 repetitions.

Modified Toe-touch With Rotation

Stand with your feet hip-width apart and bend at the waist with your forehead in the direction of your right knee. Hold for 10–15 seconds. Stand up straight again and then lower your forehead toward your left knee. Hold for 10–15 seconds. Start with three repetitions and then increase gradually by one every other day until you reach 12 repetitions.

Extension Exercises

As you become more comfortable and your back muscles begin to lengthen and strengthen, you can start extension exercises. Gravity naturally pulls the back forward and down. These exercises strengthen the muscles needed to counteract the force of gravity.

Hip Extension

Lie on your back on a table with one leg hanging over the side. Gently lower the leg from the hip toward the floor. When you feel the stretch in your hip, hold for 10 seconds. If possible, have a partner gently push on your knee to increase the stretch. Return your leg to table height. Do five repetitions and repeat with the other leg. Add stretches two at a time as this exercise becomes easier.

Reverse Sit-up

This involves working with a partner, who will have to hold down your legs. Lie on your stomach with only your legs and pelvis on a table. Keep your upper body horizontal in the air and let your hands hang down as you look at the floor. Have your partner hold your ankles while you bend down at the waist until the top of your head is pointing to the floor. Then slowly lift your upper body until it is horizontal again. Do five repetitions and add two at a time as this exercise becomes easier.

Standing Back Extension

Stand up straight with your feet hip-width apart and arms at your sides. Slowly lean your upper body back from the waist. Try to look at the ceiling. Hold for 10 seconds, then relax and straighten up. Do five repetitions and gradually add stretches two at a time as this exercise becomes easier.

Exercises for Sciatica

By doing the right back exercises the right way, you have a great chance of stopping your sciatica and back pain and keeping your back healthy and strong. Although many people may feel that bed rest is the best way for treating sciatica this is simply not true. Yes resting for a day or two can help to relieve the pain felt when the sciatica flares up but after that, because a person has become inactive, they will find that the pain actually becomes much worse.

This is because without them carrying out any kind of exercise or movement the muscles in the back and their spine will lose its condition and will then find it very difficult to support the back properly. The weakening of the back could lead to injuries and this will only then increase the amount of pain that the person is feeling.

Exercise is actually extremely important to our spine especially in order to keep the discs within the spine healthy. By carrying out movement a person is actually enable nutrients and fluids to gain access to these discs which in turn ensures that they remain fit and healthy.

Stretching exercises are especially good for treating sciatica as they target those muscles which are causing the pain because they have become tense (tight) and not as flexible as they should be. People who take up sciatica exercises find that it helps to strengthen and stretch the back muscles and they can recover much more quickly when they suffer a flare up of sciatica in the future. Plus it has also been found that it actually helps to prevent them from suffering future episodes of sciatica pain.

The most common sciatica exercises that are recommended for the treatment of sciatica related pain are the Hamstring stretching exercises.

The hamstrings are the muscles located in the back of the thigh and help in bending the knee. You must also perform exercises to strengthen the abdominal muscles in order to get relief from the sciatica pain. You can consult exercise experts or take the help of back exercise videos to learn specific exercises to relieve sciatica pain.

Even if your back already hurts, or is strained, there is a good chance that you can make it better. If you don't exercise reasonably regularly, especially as you age, the muscles supporting and surrounding your back will eventually get weak and stiff. Then these muscles won't be able to work well enough when you most need them to - when you put a strain on your back.

Things You Can Do To Help Your Back

1. Stand upright and pay attention to posture - don't slouch.

2. Sit upright at your desk with your lower back slightly curved. Don't slump in your chair or hunch over your keyboard. Set your workstation up correctly - screen at eye level.

3. Change your position frequently. Get up and walk around every 20-30 minutes even if it's only for 30 seconds.

4. Eat healthily and manage your weight. Extra weight, especially around your waist, strains your back. A simple diet with a good selection of fresh foods is one of the keys to overall health.

5. Do specific back strengthening exercises. (Find out about the Better Back System).

6. Also exercise to strengthen your stomach and 'core' muscles which help support your back.

7. Push rather than pull heavy objects. If you're lifting something heavy, use your leg muscles and hold it close to your body. Don't bend over and strain your back.

ABOUT THE AUTHOR

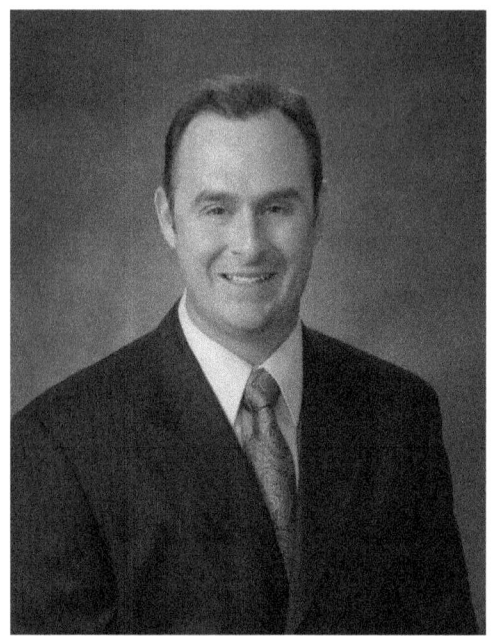

Dr. Barry Coniglio

Awarded "NJ Top Doc"

*Rated Best Chiropractic Office
in Southern New Jersey 1996-2007 &
Gloucester County 2003, 2004, 2008-2011*

- Doctorate Degree- Los Angeles College of Chiropractic

- Board Certified Chiropractic Orthopedist - National Chiropractic College

- Board Certified Sports Chiropractor - New York Chiropractic College

- Chiropractic Internship- Whittier Chiropractic Health Center

- Licensed to practice chiropractic in New Jersey and Pennsylvania

- Board Certified- American Chiropractic Association Council for Sports Injuries

- Diplomat- American Board of Chiropractic Examiners

- Board Certified- Chiropractic Orthopedics

- Member- American Chiropractic Association, Association of New Jersey Chiropractors

- Past President- Southern New Jersey Chiropractic Society

- State Board of Directors for the Association of New Jersey Chiropractors

Glossary

Abduction: Abduction refers to moving an extremity away from the body

Acute Back Pain: Back pain that lasts a short while, usually a few days to several weeks. Episodes lasting longer than three months are not considered acute

Adduction: Describes a motion that involves bringing an extremity back to the body's midline

Adult onset diabetes: Also called noninsulin-dependent, or type 2: characterized by elevated blood sugar, gradual onset, and complications involving many organ systems. The disease usually occurs in middle-aged and older adults

Allergies: Allergies are abnormal reactions of the immune system that occur in response to otherwise harmless substances

Alzheimer's Disease: A progressive, degenerative disease characterized by loss of function and death of nerve cells in several areas of the brain leading to loss of cognitive functions such as memory and language. Alzheimer's disease is the most common cause of dementia. Other causes include multiple small strokes (multi-infarct dementia), alcoholism, and less common degenerative conditions such as progressive supranuclear palsy, Pick's disease, etc.

Angina/coronary Artery Disease: Chest pain that occurs secondary to the inadequate delivery of oxygen to the heart muscle, often described as a heavy or squeezing pain in the midsternum area of the chest. Coronary artery disease is the process by which the coronary arteries become narrowed or completely occluded by cholesterol plaques. Ultimately, this is the underlying cause of angina and heart attack (myocardial infarction)

Antibody: An immunoglobulin molecule that reacts with a specific antigen that induced its synthesis and with similar molecules; classified according to mode of action as agglutinin, bacteriolysin, hemolysin, opsonins, or precipitin. Antibodies are synthesized by B lymphocytes that have been activated by the binding of an antigen to a cell-surface receptor

Applied Kinesiology: A method of testing muscle strength to detect the presence of disease, vitamin deficiency, and other problems

Aromatherapy: The use of essential oils (which are extracted from herbs, flowers, resin, woods, and roots) in body and skin care treatments is known as aromatherapy. Used as a healing technique for thousands of years by the Egyptians, Greeks, and Romans, essential oils aid in relaxation, improve circulation, and help the healing of wounds.

Arthroscopic Surgery: Arthroscopic surgery is a less-invasive procedure for surgeons to diagnose and repair joint injuries

Asthma: A disease process that is characterized by episodic, often sudden narrowing of the bronchi (lung passageways), causing wheezing, shortness of breath, chest tightness, and cough. Factors which can exacerbate asthma include rapid changes in temperature or humidity, allergies, upper respiratory infections, exercise, stress, or smoke

Atrial Fibrillation: A condition in which disorganized electrical conduction in the atria (upper chambers of the heart) results in irregular heartbeat and ineffective pumping of blood into the ventricle

Biofeedback: Biofeedback utilizes a system of sensitive instruments that relay information about the physical condition of the body. Used as a primary therapy, or in conjunction with other methods, biofeedback provides deep relaxation and stress management skills to prevent stress-related disorders and illness. These skills, including deep breathing and guided imagery, offer self-regulation and control over mental, emotional, and physical processes.

Bursitis: Bursitis is inflammation of the fluid filled sacs, bursa, that cushion areas of pressure between joints, muscles, and tendons

Cavitation: Pop that occurs in a spinal joint when vertebral surfaces (facets) are separated to create a vacuum that pulls in nitrogen gas

Cervical Vertebrae: There are seven vertebrae in the cervical or neck area of the spine

Chronic Fatigue: An illness of uncertain cause that is characterized by unexplained fatigue, weakness, muscle pain, lymph node swelling, and malaise

Chronic Pancreatitis: Chronic inflammation of the pancreas, which may be asymptomatic or symptomatic and which is due to digestion of pancreatic tissue by its own enzymes and consequent inflammation. Common causes are alcohol abuse and obstruction due to gall stones

Chronic: Describes an illness or medical condition that lasts over a long period and sometimes causes a long-term change in the body

Cirrhosis of the liver: Liver scarring causing progressive loss of function with abdominal swelling, malaise, digestive problems, and clotting disorders. Common causes include alcohol abuse and chronic viral infections

Cold Packs: Cold packs are a frozen gel substance used by physical therapists to treat areas of pain and

Complementary Therapy: Therapeutic practices which are not currently considered an integral part of conventional allopathic medical practice

Congestive Heart Failure: A condition in which ineffective pumping of the heart leads to an accumulation of fluid in the lungs and legs. Typical symptoms include shortness of breath with exertion, difficulty breathing when lying flat and leg or ankle swelling. Causes include chronic hypertension, cardiomyopathy, and myocardial infarction (heart attack)

Connective Tissue Massage: Techniques designed to specifically affect the connective tissue of the body.

Contour Analysis: Procedure in which an angled light is passed through a grid to the surface of the patient's body to produce a pattern of shadows that is viewed on a screen and/or photographed. The resultant picture resembles a topographic map

Cystic Fibrosis: A generalized disorder of infants, children, and young adults, in which there is widespread dysfunction of the exocrine glands, characterized by signs of chronic pulmonary disease (due to excess mucus production in the respiratory tract) and pancreatic deficiency. There is an ineffective immunologic defense against bacteria in the lungs. The degree of involvement of organs and glandular systems may vary greatly, with consequent variations in the clinical picture

D.C.: Abbreviation for Doctor of Chiropractic

Deep Tissue Massage: More than a deep massage, deep tissue/deep muscle massage is administered to affect the sub-layer of musculature and fascia. The muscles must be relaxed in order to effectively perform deep tissue massage, otherwise tight surface muscles prevent the practitioner from reaching deeper musculature. It helps with chronic muscular pain and injury rehabilitation, and reduces inflammation-related pain caused by arthritis and tendinitis. It is generally integrated with other massage techniques.

Degenerative: Causing or showing a gradual deterioration in the structure of a body part with a consequent loss of the part's ability to function

Depression: A mental state of depressed mood characterized by feelings of sadness, despair, and discouragement. Depression ranges from normal feelings of "the blues" through dysthymia to major depression. It in many ways resembles grief and mourning following bereavement; there are often feelings of low self-esteem, guilt and self-reproach, withdrawal from interpersonal contact and somatic symptoms such as eating and sleep disturbances

Deprivation: The act of taking something away from somebody or preventing somebody from having something

Detoxification: Detoxification is one of the more widely used treatments and concepts in alternative medicine. It is based on the principle that illnesses can be caused by the accumulation of toxic substances (toxins) in the body. Eliminating existing toxins and avoiding new toxins are essential parts of the healing process. Detoxification utilizes a variety of tests and techniques

Diabetic: Relating to or caused by diabetes, especially diabetes mellitus

DVT or Deep Vein Thrombosis: DVT refers to deep vein thrombosis, a term used to describe blood clots in the arms, and most commonly the legs

Dynamic thrust: Chiropractic adjustment delivered suddenly and forcefully to move vertebrae, often resulting in a popping sound

Dysfunction: A disturbance in the usual pattern of activity or behavior

Electrical Stimulation: Electrical Stimulation is a therapy modality used to strengthen muscles and promote healing

Emphysema and Chronic Obstructive Pulmonary Disease (COPD): A progressive disease process that most commonly results from smoking. COPD is characterized by persistent difficulty breathing, wheezing, and chronic cough. Treatment includes absolute avoidance of smoking and the use of bronchodilators and oxygen for those with advanced disease. Complications include bronchitis, recurrent pneumonia, and heart failure

Enzyme Replacement: Approach that correlates recurring "subluxation patterns" with the results of a 24-hour urinalysis so that spinal adjustments and nutritional measures can be combined

Exercise Therapy: Motion of the body or its parts to relieve symptoms or to improve function, leading to physical fitness

Extension: Extension describes the motion of increasing the angle of the joint

Fibromyalgia: An illness characterized by pain in and around joints, often with specific points of tenderness; its exact nature and cause is uncertain

Flexion: Flexion describes a movement that entails decreasing the angle of a body part

Foot Drop: Foot drop describes a condition where the ankle cannot lift the foot off the ground

Fracture: A split or division in something such as a system, organization, or agreement

Gait: Gait is a common term used by health care professionals. Learn what gait refers to and its various forms

Geriatrics: Geriatrics is the study of medicine pertaining to the elderly and disease processes of aging

Herniate: To project through a rupture in the wall of a body cavity, or through a normal or potential opening that has become enlarged

Holistic Medicine: Holistic medicine observes all aspects of a person's life; emotions, lifestyle, environment, etc. A holistic practitioner often utilizes a combination of conventional treatments along with alternative therapies. Thus, the evaluation and treatment of the persons illness including preventative intervention, cares for the whole person, remedying more than just the immediate symptoms or disease.

Hormone: A chemical secreted by an endocrine gland or some nerve cells that regulates the function of a specific tissue or organ

Hot Packs: Hot packs are a modality used by physical therapists to decrease pain due to muscle strains and spasms

Imaging: A technique, often computerized, for obtaining images of bodies or body parts for diagnosis, emergency rescue, or surveillance; the use of mental images to try to ease pain, alter the course of a disease, or help in achieving a goal

Impotence (erectile dysfunction or ED): Partial or complete inability to achieve and/or maintain erection, which may be intermittent or persistent and arises from a variety of causes. Its frequency increases with age, certain diseases, and the use of a wide variety of prescription medications

Infection: The reproduction and proliferation of microorganisms within the body

Infertility: Partial or complete inability for a couple to achieve pregnancy. There are a number of causes, some inherent in the man, some in the woman, and some in various incompatibilities between the two

Inflammatory bowel diseases (Crohn's and ulcerative colitis): Inflammatory diseases of the gastrointestinal tract that seem to have both genetic and environmental causes, not well understood. The peak incidence of the onset of these diseases is between 15 and 25 years of age. Crohn's also occurs in later years between the ages of 55 and 60. Common symptoms include recurrent abdominal pains, fever, nausea, vomiting, weight loss, and diarrhea which are occasionally bloody. Complications include gastrointestinal bleeding, fistulas, and anal fissures

Insomnia: Inability to fall asleep or to remain asleep long enough to feel rested, especially when this is a problem that continues over time

Integrative Medicine: Alternative and conventional (allopathic) methodologies are combined to stimulate healing or the resolution of the disease.

Integrative/ Eclectic Massage: Combines various massage, bodywork, and somatic therapy techniques utilized by a practitioner in the course of a session.

Intervertebral Disc: The tough cartilage that serves as a cushion between two vertebrae. Each disk has a gelatinous-like center (nucleus pulposus) that may protrude to form a disk herniation

Isometrics and Muscle Balancing: Isometric Muscle Balancing is based on the muscle testing positions used in kinesiology. Balancing and strengthening the 42 major muscles are accomplished by isometric action, producing a feeling of lightness and an increase in energy. A 45-minute to one hour session also includes instruction in creating and maintaining balance and proper postural habits, as well as attention to diet and attitude.

Juvenile onset diabetes: Also called insulin-dependent, or type 1: characterized by elevated blood sugar, insulin deficiency, sudden onset, severe hyperglycemia, rapid progression to ketoacidosis, and death unless treated with insulin. The disease may occur at any age, but is most common in childhood or adolescence

Ligament: A sheet or band of tough fibrous tissue that connects bones or cartilage at a joint or supports an organ, muscle, or other body part

Locked Spinal Joint: Sudden binding that occurs when two joint surfaces are shifted out of their normal alignment by an awkward movement that triggers muscle spasm

Low-Force Technique: Use of an adjusting machine and/or reflex technique said to be an alternative to forceful manipulation ("dynamic thrust")

Lumbar Vertebrae: The five bones in the lower-back portion of the spine

Lumbosacral Strain: Strain or injury of joints or ligaments at the base of the spine where the last lumbar vertebra (L5) is connected to the sacrum. Strain or disk degeneration in this area is probably the most common cause of low-back pain

Lung Disease: A group of lung disorders which result in scarring and dysfunction of the alveoli (air sacs) in the lung. This results in poor oxygen diffusion from the air into the bloodstream. Widespread inflammation in the lung leads to fibrosis (scarring). Causes include chronic exposure to organic and inorganic dusts, fumes, vapors, radiation, medications, and certain lung infections. Examples include asbestosis, silicosis, coal worker's pneumoconiosis, and diffuse interstitial fibrosis. Smoking increases the risk in all cases

Lupus: A systemic autoimmune disease. Individuals with lupus produce antibodies to their own body tissues. The resultant inflammation can cause kidney damage, arthritis, pericarditis, and vasculitis

Maintenance Care: Subluxation-based program of periodic spinal examinations and adjustments to help maintain health

Manual Lymphatic Drainage: The strokes applied in manual lymph drainage are intended to stimulate the movement of the lymphatic fluids in order to assist the body in cleansing. This is a gentle, rhythmical technique that cleanses the connective tissue of inflammatory materials and toxins, enhances the activity of the immune system, reduces pain, and lowers the activity of the sympathetic nervous system.

Massage: Massage is the practice of applying structured pressure, tension, motion, or vibration — manually or with mechanical aids — to the soft tissues of the body, including muscles, connective tissue, tendons, ligaments, joints and lymphatic vessels, to achieve a therapeutic response. Massage can be applied to all parts of the body or successively to the whole body, to heal injury, relieve psychological stress, manage pain, and improve circulation.

Medical Massage: Performing medical massage requires a firm background in pathology and utilizes specific treatments appropriate to working with disease, pain, and recovery from injury..

Migraine: A throbbing headache that usually affects only one side of the head. Nausea, vomiting, increased sensitivity to light, and other symptoms often accompany migraine

Mobilization: Method of manipulation, movement, or stretching to increase range of motion in muscles and joints that does not involve a high-velocity thrust

Motion Palpation: Useful method of locating fixations and loss of mobility in the spine by feeling the motion of specific spinal segments as the patient moves

MRI: An imaging technique that uses electromagnetic radiation to obtain images of the body's soft tissues, e.g. the brain and spinal cord. The body is subjected to a powerful magnetic field, allowing tiny signals from atomic nuclei to be detected and then processed and converted into images by a computer

Multiple Sclerosis: Neurodegenerative disease characterized by the gradual accumulation of focal plaques of demyelination particularly in the brain and spinal cord, producing disparate symptoms (for example, visual disturbances, muscle weakness, and bladder problems)

Musculoskeletal: Referring to structures involving tendons, muscles, ligaments, and joints

Nerve Root: One of the two nerve bundles emerging from the spinal cord that joins to form a segmental spinal nerve

Nerve: A bundle of fibers forming a network that transmits messages in the form of impulses between the brain or spinal cord and the body's organs. Motor nerves carry impulses outward to the muscles and glands, while sensory nerves carry inbound information about the body's movements and sensations. Mixed nerves perform both functions

Neurology: Neurology is the medical science of the nervous system

Neuromuscular Therapy: Neuromuscular therapy (NMT) is a significant methodology for assessing, treating and preventing soft tissue injuries and chronic pain. NMT, a series of manual treatment protocols based on the practitioner's skill, anatomy knowledge and precise palpatory application, has found its home, not only in the treatment rooms of massage therapy, but also in occupational and physical therapy, nursing, chiropractic, osteopathic and physical medicine clinics worldwide.

Neuropathy: A disease or disorder, especially a degenerative one, which affects the nervous system

Non-force Technique: Various reflex techniques and muscle-treatment methods that do not involve forceful manipulation

Numbness: Unable to feel or have sensations, e.g. as a result of extreme cold or the application of a local anesthetic

Orthopedic Massage: Orthopedic massage integrates 10 or more modalities to treat soft tissue pain and injury. Emphasis is placed on understanding both the injury and its rehabilitation criteria. Three basic elements adhered to, despite the technical diversity in treatment, are assessment, matching the treatment to the injury, and adaptability of treatment.

Osteoporosis: Metabolic disorder associated with fractures of the femoral neck, vertebrae, and distal forearm. It occurs commonly in women within 15-20 years after menopause, and is caused by factors associated with menopause including estrogen deficiency. It also occurs in men, perhaps associated with testosterone deficiency; and in persons treated with chronic steroids, and those with vitamin D deficiency, hyperparathyroidism, hyperthyroidism, alcoholism, and cigarette smoking

Parkinsonism: A progressive, neurological disease first described in 1817 by James Parkinson. Characteristic symptoms include a slow tremor of extremities and head, rigidity, and gait disturbances

Peptic Ulcer Disease: An ulcer in the wall of the stomach or duodenum resulting from the digestive action of the gastric juice on the mucous membrane when the latter is rendered susceptible to its action. Most commonly caused by anti-inflammatory medications or infection with Helicobacter pylori; in older persons, stomach cancer causes a significant proportion of cases

Peripheral: Near the surface of an organ or the body; at the edge or end

Physical Fitness: A state of well-being in which performance is optimal, often as a result of physical conditioning which may be prescribed for disease therapy

Physical Therapy: The auxiliary health profession which makes use of physical therapy techniques to prevent, correct, and alleviate movement dysfunction of anatomic or physiologic origin

Pituitary: Relating to or produced by the pituitary gland

Plantar Fasciitis: Plantar fasciitis is an inflammation of the plantar fascia that runs from the heel bone in the foot to the toes

Predisposition: A liability or tendency to do something such as behave in a particular way

Pregnancy Massage/Prenatal Massage: Prenatally, specific techniques can reduce pregnancy discomforts and concerns and enhance the physiological and emotional well-being of both mother and fetus. Skilled, appropriate touch facilitates labor, shortening labor times and easing pain and anxiety. In the postpartum period, specialized techniques rebalance structure, physiology, and emotions of the new mother, and may help her to bond with and care for her infant. Specialized, advanced training in the anatomy, physiology, complications, precautions, and contraindications is highly recommended, and many practitioners request referrals from physicians prior to therapy. (Click Here see research on Pregnancy) massage

Proprioception: Proprioception is the term that refers to the ability to determine the orientation of one's arm or leg in the air

Radicular Pain: Radicular pain is often due to disc herniation. Find out what "radicular" means in this glossary overview

Reflex Analysis: A testing procedure in which diagnoses are made by testing muscle strength while placing manual pressure on alleged "reflex points"

Reflex Sympathetic Dystrophy: Reflex sympathetic dystrophy is a condition of increased sympathetic discharge in an extremity that often occurs after trauma

REM: Jerky movements of the eyeballs while the eyes are closed, characteristic of somebody who is dreaming while asleep, especially during REM sleep

Rheumatoid Arthritis: Chronic inflammatory disease in which there is deformation and destruction of joints. Generally considered by some to be an autoimmune disorder in which immune complexes are formed in joints and excite an inflammatory response

RICE- Rest, Ice Compression, and Elevation: RICE is a commonly used acronym for the management of acute soft tissue injuries. Discover the meaning behind these letters so that you can use this treatment if necessary

Sacrum: The triangular bone that serves as a base for the spinal column and connects the pelvic bones

Sciatica: Pain and tenderness extending from the back of the hip down to the calf, usually caused by a protrusion of vertebral disk substance pressing on the roots of the sciatic nerve

Seizure: A sudden attack or convulsion due to involuntary electrical activity in the brain. It can result in a wide variety of symptoms, such as: muscle twitches, staring, tongue biting, urination, loss of consciousness and total body shaking. Examples include: focal seizure, absence seizure, partial seizure, psychomotor seizure, petit-mal seizure and grand-mal seizure

Sickle Cell Disease: Common in races of people from areas in which malaria is endemic. The cause is a mutation in the gene that codes for one of the components (the beta chain) of hemoglobin. This mutation makes red blood cells change from the normal discoid shape to a sickle shape when the oxygen tension is low. These sickled cells become trapped in capillaries or damaged in transit, leading to severe anemia, pain in joints, bones, and other parts of the body, skin ulcers, etc

Soft Tissue Release: Soft tissue release (STR) is a powerful injury treatment technique developed in Europe with the world's fastest sprinters. Due to the amazing amounts of prize money and endorsement contracts available to these athletes, faster and more permanent results were warranted. STR was developed to meet this need. Recovery rates once considered impossible by traditional therapists and sports medicine doctors were achieved. These are not new concepts, but are based on European osteopathy techniques, along with insights from quantum physics. In recent years, STR has been given clinical application for chronic low back pain and whiplash injuries.

STR deals directly with the reasons for soft tissue dysfunctions and subsequent referred pain and nerve entrapment. In acute conditions, STR affects the insidious way scar tissue is formed, and in chronic conditions STR breaks up the fibrotic and adhered mass of scar tissue to quickly allow the muscle to return to its natural resting length. Once the muscle or muscle group has returned to the original resting length, there is an immediate release from the pain induced by the inflammation response.

With STR, the client is placed in a particular position so that the muscle begins to stretch in a very specific direction or plane. The exact location of the injury has been defined and a determined pressure is applied directly into the affected tissue or along a specific line of injury. At the same time, depending whether passive or active techniques are being used, the client is given a set of instructions that now engage the antagonist of the muscles involved. The muscle is extended from a fixed position in a determined direction under a pinpoint of pressure.

Decrease in pain and increase in range of motion are often immediate, offsetting any minor discomfort experienced. STR can be modified so there is no client discomfort at all. The flowing motions of STR and total client control afford new levels of deep tissue work and subsequent pain relief.

Spasticity: Spasticity is a condition in which certain muscles are continuously contracted

Spinal Adjustment: A chiropractic term that most chiropractors use to describe methods used to correct spinal problems, whether by hand or with an instrument

Spinal Manipulation: A forceful, high-velocity thrust that stretches a joint beyond its passive range of movement in order to increase its mobility. Manipulation is usually accompanied by an audible pop or click.

Spondylolisthesis: Spondylolisthesis occurs when anterior displacement of a vertebra or the vertebral column in relation to the vertebrae below occurs

Sports massage: Sports massage consists of specific components designed to reduce injuries, alleviate inflammation, provide warm-up, etc. for amateur and professional athletes before, during, after, and within their training regimens.

Sprain: A sprain refers an injury sustained to a ligament in the body

Stenosis: A constriction or narrowing of a duct, passage, or opening in the body

Stress: The body's normal response to anything that disturbs its natural physical, emotional, or mental balance. Stress reduction refers to various strategies that counteract this response and produce a sense of relaxation and tranquility

Stroke: A condition due to impaired blood flow causing lack of oxygen to part of the brain which may lead to reversible or irreversible damage. Depending on the area of the brain that is damaged, a stroke can cause coma, paralysis, speech problems, and/or dementia

Stroke: A stroke is also known as a cva, or cerebrovascular accident. Learn more about the definition of stroke in this glossary

Structure: A system or organization made up of interrelated parts functioning as a whole

Subluxation: The medical definition is incomplete or partial dislocation—a condition, visible on x-ray films, in which the bony surfaces of a joint no longer face each other exactly but remain partially aligned

Surface Electromyography (SEMG): A procedure that measures skin temperature and electrical activity in muscles surrounding the spine

Syndrome: A group of signs and symptoms that together is characteristic or indicative of a specific disease or other disorder

Tendon: An inelastic cord or band of tough white fibrous connective tissue that attaches a muscle to a bone or other part

Tendonitis: Tendonitis is an inflammatory condition that affects the tissue that connects muscle to bones. Read about this term here

TENS: A TENS unit stands for transcutaneous electrical nerve stimulation. It is a small battery operated machine used by physical therapists to decrease pain

Thermography: A diagnostic procedure that images heat from body surfaces

Thoracic Vertebrae: There are twelve vertebrae in the thoracic or upper-back portion of the spine

Thyroid: Relating to, situated in, or secreted by the thyroid gland

Tingling: To feel a sensation of stinging, pricking, or vibration, e.g. from cold or a slight electric shock, or cause somebody to feel this

Trigger Point: A trigger point is a taught band of muscle that can refer pain to various parts of the body

Trimester: A period of three months, especially one of the three three-month periods into which human pregnancy is divided for medical purposes

Tumor: An uncontrolled growth or mass of body cells, which may be malignant or benign and has no physiological function

Ultrasound: Ultrasound machines are a treatment modality used by physical therapists that utilize high or low frequency sound wave

Vertebra: Bony segment of the spine that encircles and helps protect the spinal cord and nerves. The plural of vertebra is vertebrae

Vertebrae: A bone of the spinal column, typically consisting of a thick body, a bony arch enclosing a hole for the spinal cord, and stubby projections that connect with adjacent bones

Vertebral Artery: Arteries, one on each side, that thread through holes in the six upper cervical vertebrae